HypnoBirthing®
The Mongan Method

HypnoBirthing®
The Mongan Method

The breakthrough approach to safer,
easier, comfortable birthing

Fourth Edition
Marie F. Mongan, M.Ed., M.Hy.

Souvenir Press

NOTE: The HypnoBirthing Institute and this book describing HypnoBirthing methods and techniques are not intended to represent an anatomically and medically precise overview of pregnancy and birth, nor are they designed to represent medical advice or a prescription for medical procedure. The content of this book is the accumulation of the author's philosophical thought on birth, her experience in attending births, her research, and her opinion, along with that of others. It is not intended to replace the advice of a medical doctor. It is advisable for any pregnant woman to seek the advice of a licensed/certified health care provider before undertaking any pregnancy- or labour-related programme.

Persons following any course of action recommended or described in this book or within HypnoBirthing classes do so of their own free will. The author, the publisher, and the HypnoBirthing Institute assume no responsibility for any possible complication related to either the pregnancy or the labour of the participant.

Copyright © 1992, 1998, 2005, 2015 by Marie F. Mongan

First published in the USA by Health Communications, Inc.

First published in Great Britain in 2007 by Souvenir Press Ltd.
Reprinted 2007, 2008 (twice), 2009 (twice), 2010 (twice),
2011 (twice), 2012, 2013 (twice), 2014, 2015

This fourth and expanded edition first published in Great Britain in 2016
by Souvenir Press Ltd, 43 Great Russell Street, London WC1B 3PD

Reprinted 2017, 2018

The right of Marie F. Mongan to be identified as
the author of this work has been asserted in accordance
with the Copyright, Designs and Patents Act, 1988

Inside book design by Lawna Patterson Oldfield
Illustrations by Paul Svancara

ISBN   9780285643352

Typeset by M Rules

Printed and bound by Nørhaven, Denmark

This Fourth Edition of HypnoBirthing,
the Mongan Method, is dedicated to those many
genuinely caring birth professionals—doctors, nurses, nurse midwives,
Certified Professional Midwives, childbirth educators, and doulas—
who have witnessed the beauty of HypnoBirthing and
who have seen it with open eyes, open minds, and open hearts,
and who have then moved forward to bring calm and gentle
birthing into the lives of the parents they serve and
the colleagues with whom they work.

"Women have access to an unstoppable energy that transcends fear and negativity. Women who tap into that energy have the power not only to achieve their own life purpose and goals; but using their personal stories as a template, they inspire other women to do the same—to go beyond what they ever thought was possible."

—**Patricia Jocelyn**
Author, Journalist, Spiritual Lecturer

Contents

Foreword

Marie Mongan is a woman who has devoted her entire life to working with women of all ages and in all walks of life. Through her book and the HypnoBirthing Method, she shares the conviction of her own personal birthing experience and her sensitivity to the emotional and spiritual needs of birthing women. The message about the normality of birth that this book delivers is an essential one for all families who believe in and care about birthing their babies in safety, calm, and peace.

This book, and the HypnoBirthing program itself, has provided me, and other doctors who share a belief in normal birth, a framework within which to practise obstetrics in the manner in which our education has qualified us and in the direction in which our hearts have led us. It has changed the way many of us practise obstetrics.

I began "delivering" babies in 1983. I believed in the use of drugs to manage obstetrical pain. In spite of my best efforts to use good sound medical judgment, I saw lots of complications, including babies with compromised breathing. I believed that epidurals were a medical blessing for labouring mothers. I had a 25 percent C-section rate.

Many patients demanded natural births. I then performed hundreds of deliveries using pushing and blowing while holding off analgesics until the mother could no longer take the pain. I saw babies that were no longer respiratorily compromised, but both mother and baby were exhausted. Quite often there was a need for respiratory support with oxygen. But my C-section rate had fallen to 5 percent.

Next, I used visualisation and guided imagery with patients to manage pain. On occasion, I still had to use narcotics and a rare epidural. I continued to see exhausted babies who were not fully able to bond. I still had a C-section rate of 5 percent.

Eventually, I began using hypnosis to manage pain during birth. The results were okay. Babies were less often compromised and very rarely needed oxygen; but mothers still experienced painful births. My C-section rate remained at 5 percent.

A few years ago, I made the transition to HypnoBirthing, and I now truly believe that normal birthing does not have to involve pain. I have attended over 200 births of women who prepared for birth by learning and using the techniques and philosophy of HypnoBirthing—"The Mongan Method." All of the families have left their birthings excited about the birth event. I see support people meaningfully involved with the mother and assisting in many different ways. I have had no complications. No babies have needed oxygen or any support other than warming by mother's body. My C-section count is three—in as many years. I have given absolutely no analgesic drugs since I began using HypnoBirthing with mothers.

Over the years, I have come to realise that during a birthing, I no longer perform "deliveries"; I attend and observe as mothers birth their babies in calm and comfort, and birthing companions receive the babies as they emerge. It is as if my new role is to be present to witness the miracle of HypnoBirthing.

Now I enthusiastically lecture to medical groups on a regular basis about the merits of HypnoBirthing as a means of achieving easier, more comfortable births for labouring mothers. I am more than happy to talk to health-care professionals (or anyone else) about my experiences with truly natural birthing. I have a large number of happy HypnoBirthing families—mothers and fathers—who love to talk about their own birthing experiences.

In my position as a faculty member of the Atlanta Family Medicine Residency Program in Atlanta, Georgia, I trained medical residents to use HypnoBirthing as an option for the families they will serve.

I heartily recommend this book, and the well-thought-out program that it accompanies, for its contribution toward making the birth of our children a positive and gentle step on the way to a better world.

Lorne R. Campbell, Sr., M.D.
Clinical Professor, Family Medicine

Looking Back Over 25 Years

W hen the publisher of the third edition of our HypnoBirthing textbook invited me to write a revision of the book for our 25th anniversary, it opened up a flood of memories and thoughts about the journey that has brought HypnoBirthing to where it is today. Mongan Method HypnoBirthing is the leader and most comprehensive natural and instinctive birth education programme that exists. It has, from the very beginning, reached beyond simple relaxation and introduced many advanced hypnosis techniques into the birthing classroom. The coincidence of this being our 25th anniversary year called back thoughts of experiences that bubbled over in my mind and could not be quieted. Where have we been and where have we gone in a whole quarter century?

At this time 25 years ago, Maura, my daughter for whom the programme was developed, had just given birth to our grandbaby Kyle. The other two women who also prepared for their births with HypnoBirthing were due to birth at any moment. The success of Maura's birthing had the hospital staff talking about that woman in Room 201, who had no epidural, had soft music playing, and the room dimmed all through her labour. One of the nurses on duty that day, Pat, who was also pregnant, made it a point to step into Maura's room quite regularly. Each time she just stood by the door with a quizzical look on her face and stared at Maura. On one visit, she spoke, "And she hasn't had anything for pain? Really?"

I remember leaving the room briefly to get a tuna fish sandwich (usually a poor choice with a birthing mother); and when I returned, I found a midwife on her knees writing the name of the artist on the tape that was in the tape player that I had placed obscurely on the floor behind a chair.

When Maura's birth was complete, Nurse Pat came back into the room and asked for an appointment with me. As she left, she told the other nurses, "Hey, girls, this is the way I'm having my baby." My excitement doubled.

I went home that afternoon, and with my notes taken during Maura's pregnancy and her birth, I began to set down the philosophy of birth that had been waiting all these many years since I was a child. One by one, I started to expand on the chapters of the coil-bound book I had prepared for my first three pioneer mums. I knew that I needed to put these feelings and observations down so that they could be shared with others. Writing that book was the easiest thing I've ever done. My enthusiasm was at peak, and my mind just wouldn't shut down for anything.

With the other two births happening on the heels of the first, and followed by Nurse Pat's birth, HypnoBirthing became a buzzword in that hospital. Soon a number of curious hypnotherapists, who heard about what was happening in Concord, New Hampshire, called to ask, "Will you teach me what you taught Maura about birthing with hypnosis?" In no time, there were a number of hypnotherapists meeting with eager couples. The National Guild of Hypnotists invited me to present the programme at their annual educational convention, and then we were on our way. Simply by word of mouth, we had HypnoBirthings occurring all over the country.

A Paradigm Shift Began

There we were. I began to receive so many calls that I started to teach classes. Pregnant mothers and their birth companions filled the parent classes, and hypnotherapists, nurses, and doulas came to become practitioners.

I had no idea of how urgently pregnant women were craving a better way to birth than the standard births that were offered by hospitals. They were hungry for a programme that would allow them to forego anaesthesia, but at the same time, make it possible for them to birth gently and in comfort. Since most hospital personnel themselves did not believe that birth could be free of fear and pain, there was only the home birth route, which also bore the burden of lack of public recognition and a lot of misinformation.

I found out quickly when NBC's TV show *Dateline* presented a full-hour feature on birthing with hypnosis. At the end of the show, hundreds of people called or wrote to producers to tell them that they had neglected to tell the public that the programme is HypnoBirthing. The following morning there was a front-page article on the MSNBC website about HypnoBirthing, stating that it was I who founded the programme. They gave a link directly to our HypnoBirthing website. Without a bit of exaggeration, I can honestly say that we received almost 5,000 calls and emails over the next few weeks.

HypnoBirthing took on a life of its own, and in a very short time, it took over my life as well. All of a sudden we needed staff to be able to give referrals from a referral system we didn't even have as yet. We needed a second telephone and another person to receive the calls. We stepped beyond the realm of a passion and into the realm of business. A business we hadn't planned for.

It looked as though the change in the way birth was viewed by the general public, and care providers as well, would come easily. With the impetus of that NBC show behind us, we saw a large number of pregnant families flocking to our classes. It became increasingly obvious, however, that not many care providers were impressed.

When I first started teaching and accompanying birthing families into the hospital those many years ago, I remember naively thinking that surely doctors and midwives would be pulling me out of birthing rooms to inquire how they could replicate those beautiful scenes. I was sure that once they witnessed a few HypnoBirthing mothers breathing their babies down to crowning in deep relaxation, they would insist on having all of their mums know how to achieve this phenomenon. I waited. The nurses were enthusiastic, and several midwives joined our ranks. Doctors regularly commented on how "remarkable" the births were, but except for a few, they showed no curiosity as to how these results were achieved. Even though they saw it happening time and time again, they seemed to dismiss the birthings as flukes.

In looking back now, I must admit—the acceptance of HypnoBirthing didn't come the way I thought it would. It was a very steep uphill climb. A few times a doctor would inquire, "What did you say this is?" Many saw, and frequently complimented, the birth mother on her beautiful labour. Most had no questions, however, and were not interested in knowing how more of the mothers they were caring for could birth in this way.

They quickly dismissed what they had just proclaimed "really remarkable." They were content to move on to the next room and suggest a membranes rupture or even a Pitocin drip if the mother was not progressing in line with the Friedman Curve. Pitocin was usually the order of the day if the doctor's shift was to end in a few hours. So often a beautiful calm birthing was given over to manipulation, with little thought to the dramatic change in the mother's comfort level.

Once in a while, a doctor would ask me how I could prove that what we teach in HypnoBirthing classes resulted in what we were seeing. I was always amused by that question. It reminded me of the trial scene from the movie *Chicago*, when the defence attorney is asked for evidence of something he had just brilliantly illustrated. The defence attorney replied, "And what is it that you are seeing that you need evidence of?"

Though our success didn't happen overnight, as I reflect on those years, I realise that we gradually made some significant changes just from our requests. In the hospital in Concord, New Hampshire, where HypnoBirthing first "caught on," as a mother was settling into her birthing room, her nurse would pull a chair over to the side of the bed and ask to spend a few minutes with the family so that, ". . . I can be sure that I understand exactly what you mean by some of your birth preferences."

Over time, we would find that there was already a birth ball in the room, and the nurse would remind the mother to ask when she was ready to use the tub. Someone cared enough to assure the mother that she was welcome and her requests would be honoured as far as possible. The nurses' overt support made up for the oblivion of some of the other care providers. Eventually, there were some doctors who displayed approval, but they were closet enthusiasts.

Soon I began to receive invitations from places all over the world to bring certification workshops to their countries. Canada was the first, but not far behind were the Virgin Islands, the UK, and Australia, and on and on. Over the years we have had the pleasure of training some of the finest people in the world—our teaching practitioners, without whom HypnoBirthing may have remained simply the talk of the Concord Hospital staff for a few short days; and then it would have just faded away. Those who shared our belief gravitated to our programme. It was they who truly catapulted HypnoBirthing to the position it holds today as the leader in the field of childbirth education with hypnosis.

Prior to that time, the midwives who were teaching instinctive birthing had no instructional programme or key techniques to build upon. Many of these women came in droves, as did many nurses who were discouraged with what they were seeing happening in hospitals. Nancy Wainer, midwife extraordinaire and author of two books on natural birthing, joined our ranks and declared, "HypnoBirthing is the missing link we have all been seeking for years." With so many birth advocates sharing the same vision, HypnoBirthing grew. It became exemplary of what gentle birth should look like and what it should feel like for the birthing mother and baby. In addition to seeing what HypnoBirthing could do for the families, these birth professionals also realised how it brought more ease and joy to their own work. Nurses who saw instinctive birthing and worked with HypnoBirthing families were instrumental in bringing HypnoBirthing to their hospitals' education programmes.

It was a good fit, in spite of those who found it difficult to believe that a baby could descend and emerge without his mother scrunching up her body, holding her breath, and forcefully pushing her baby out with all her might. Even now, a whole quarter of a century later, there are people who still subscribe to "purple pushing." It's what is portrayed in movies and on television. The general public watches and accepts, and pregnant mothers cringe.

For a long time some birthing professionals tenaciously clung to almost gymnastic-like moves that had the mum pulling on a rolled sheet or hanging over a squat bar for endless periods of time. Some facilities had women hanging upright from a huge knot in a rope "to use the benefit of gravity." Eventually that all went by the wayside with only a few continuing to preach the inevitability of severe pain. Those few sometimes even felt the need to advise the birthing mother that HypnoBirthing may work at the beginning, but not later when the pain is more severe. They were oblivious to the fact that every word they spoke instilled more fear into the minds of vulnerable mothers.

The many positive features and benefits of this shift in birthing paradigm continued to draw the attention of health-care providers. We began to see more standard health-care providers supporting HypnoBirthing families with relaxed protocols and fewer unnecessary "precautions" being applied to women who are free of special circumstances.

The light shining upon HypnoBirthing became broader and brighter. Major television morning shows and leading publications printed feature articles. Local TV channels featured our birth stories on their evening news shows. Consumers were asking about natural, instinctive birthing. It was catching on among birthing parents.

Others came and trained, and intentionally copied, and imitated. They took our concept, our materials, and our trade name; and they started their own HypnoBirthing programmes. We knew then that we had a good thing, and that good thing continued to grow.

In so many places, over the years, we saw a sizeable shift away from traditional "standard" hospital birth scenes that had women tethered with epidurals, needles, IV poles, tubes, wires, and belts. These confining and frightening scenes began to be replaced with scenes of quiet and calm women, who were free to move about or just relax. The only wires that were anywhere near were those of the earphones that mothers used to listen to soothing birthing music and scripts. In some places, women requesting calm birth were no longer restricted from eating. Care providers came to see and recognise that when endorphins are present and the constrictor hormone catecholamine is not, digestion is not arrested because the mother's body is not in the state of alarm.

HypnoBirthing gained more attention. Requests for speaking engagements and interviews poured in, along with invitations to conduct training workshops for practitioners. The HypnoBirthing way of birth was catching on.

Working on this book revision has made me realise how successful natural birth advocates have been in bringing about substantial improvements in the birthing experiences of thousands of happy birthing families, most of whom chose HypnoBirthing to prepare for their babies' births. The concept of instinctive birth also attracted the attention of some of the kindest and most caring birth professionals, nurses, doctors, and midwives who were at first curious but are today more willing to openly support instinctive birth.

When we look at trends in birthing over the past two-plus decades, we see that, truly, new life and birth are celebrated in many mainstream health-care facilities, as well as in complementary settings. This shift also points to a vast increase in the number of birth centres that have opened their doors to couples seeking natural birth but wanting a homelike atmosphere. Home births are regularly considered an option by families of all kinds of life styles—from several Hollywood movie stars and well-known entertainers and sports celebrities to families in small towns and farmlands. Many hospitals are accommodating families who are seeking an environment where they can birth naturally yet have the comfort of medical staff on hand.

Throughout the world, birth is seen as the important transformational human experience that it is. It is far more than the "process" of getting baby born and just moving on. It is recognised and celebrated in various ways. I'm told there is a large hospital in Southern California that has an entire fourth floor devoted to ABC—"A Better Childbirth."

I visited a hospital outside of Detroit that has furnished their natural birth rooms with queen beds and a homelike atmosphere with soft light and soft music—no frightening apparatus visible.

In a hospital in Minnesota, the carpeting leading into the birthing centre has inlaid appliques of dragonflies, bees, lily pads, frogs, and flowers. The rooms look like five-star hotel rooms, and there is not a visible piece of equipment in the room that shouts "Be warned!" and "Be afraid!!" I asked where some of the usual machinery and equipment is. I was told, "Right around the corner, concealed, where it belongs unless we need it, when it takes only a couple of seconds to get it." Outside is a lovely walking path lined with flowers (in the summer) and benches for couples who want to spend some of their labour time outdoors in nature. (The surgical unit has a similar "healing garden.") When a baby is born in this hospital, strains of Brahms' Lullaby filters through the sound system, and patients and visitors alike honour the new life that has just come into the world.

I once attended a birth with a mother who was the first HypnoBirthing mother at that hospital. I met a doctor by the name of Dr. Care. When he left the room, I commented to the nurse, "What a fantastic name for a person who attends births." Shortly after a young doctor walked in and the nurse said to him, "When Dr. Care was here, Mrs. Mongan commented that she thought the name Care was a perfect name for an obstetrician." The doctor extended his hand and said, "I'm happy to see my first HypnoBirthing. By the way, my name is Dr. Luti, and in Italian it means 'care.'" We all laughed. After the baby was born, the mother was told that the nurse had to take the baby away to put the bands on. The doctor looked up and said, "Bring the bands to the baby." And the mother continued to hold her newborn baby in her arms. I am sure you can guess that this mother's birth story was a beautiful one. That is all it took to start a new trend in that hospital.

Fifteen years ago, I was invited to bring the first HypnoBirthing Certification Workshop to London to train practitioners. I taught the class at St. Thomas Hospital, Florence Nightingale's hospital. This gave me the opportunity to observe and learn much about the midwifery model—an extremely mother-baby friendly model of birthing. What I saw was a birth model that is strikingly different from what I was accustomed to in the States. I liked what I saw; and I learned a great deal about this exemplary birth model that is among the most common of approaches to maternity care in the world. And a trend was begun at the hospital.

With the help of a few midwives who became HypnoBirthing practitioners early on, we were able to blend the two philosophies into the book that is now used by practitioners in the UK. The birthing unit at St. Thomas is staffed by a group of midwives whose enthusiasm for natural birth matches their gentle and friendly manner.

In a hospital in New Hampshire where a large number of Hypno-Birthing families choose to birth, the family is treated to a beautiful dinner delivered to their room on a dinner cart as elegant as one would find with room service in an upscale hotel. This hospital also has tubs in a separate room. Post-partum rooms are furnished with a trundle bed for a sibling and a queen bed for the new parents. Their infant not only rooms in, but sleeps with his parents in a family bed with a special little bed frame for the baby to safely sleep.

For healthy mothers who present minimal risk, routine practices, protocols, and procedures are being relaxed. As more couples are requesting natural birthing, more hospitals are feeding their mums.

In some places where low-risk mothers are active and mobile, they have shed the dull, ill-fitting patient gowns for attractive labour gowns for this special event. The gown is especially designed to be hospital friendly, with a halter top that ties or snaps at the back of the neck for ease of breastfeeding and strategically placed openings in the front of the gown to allow for easy access when checking baby's well-being or for birth. These facilities are but a few of the places where the shift is taking place. There are many more, and more will follow. As parents begin to make their wishes known and are willing to seek out the right environment and the right birth professionals, they are able to achieve the kind of birth that leaves them feeling fulfilled and joyful.

These hospitals are only a few of the medical facilities where the shift has taken place; and birthing families are treated as if they and their births matter. There are many more where staff has seen gentle births, and they are welcoming parents wishing this birth style. Hospitals are adjusting, and it is clear that their services are not only for the birthing families whose pregnancies are at risk. There is much hope for those parents who want natural birth but also feel more comfortable in a hospital environment.

An Opposite Paradigm Shift Appears

During these same years while natural birth advocates were basking in the growing success of an increased awareness of natural instinctive birth, a second paradigm from within the medical community appeared to be going unequivocally in a direction that is opposite from calm, gentle birthing.

This shift supports an increasing number of inductions, often scheduled ahead of the estimated delivery date (EDD) for nothing more than the chronology of the matter. Many women are being told, not advised or given a suggestion, that if they have not gone into labour before their estimated date, they will be induced on that date. This is all in spite of the fact that the EDD is just that—an estimated date. Statistics show that first-time mums average 41.3 weeks of gestation. There is little or no room within this shift for consideration of a normal, natural birth. This model feeds on suspicions and fear of "impending danger." Very early on mothers are being told of some possible danger and advised that they should expect an early induction or a C-section. Parental wishes, emotions, and expectations are swept under the rug in favour of chemical, chronological, and technological factors.

In recent years, we are hearing of exceptionally large numbers of women who are suspected of having "dangerous complications." These possible complications will necessitate regimented and strict protocols. Labour usually will call for frequent interruptions and examinations. Overuse of technology and apparatus make it almost impossible to experience normal birth. The natural rhythm and flow of labour is destroyed, and, as a result, labour can often go awry, along with the parent's dream and excitement. There seems to be a disregard for the relevance of parental input. Advocates of this shift appear to have a disregard for the sanctity of birth and do not view birth as one of the most important of our human life rituals.

These unnecessary distractions that are part of this other birth paradigm are puzzling and quite discouraging to natural birth advocates.

Their existence speaks volumes about the need to move away from the one-size-fits-all approach to birthing. It points out a screaming need for birth professionals to take a good look at the people they serve. In this way, they can begin to see and to meet birthing mothers as whole people who are experiencing a once-in-a-lifetime family event that is unlike any other. Birth touches the emotions, the spirit, and the psyche of all involved. It calls for birth professionals who are kind, caring, and sensitive. One doctor in California describes the ideal birth attendant as one who loves babies, loves birthing women, and loves birth.

As we approach the end of this first 25-year period, it becomes clear that birthing parents who choose to learn and become prepared to experience a relaxed, natural birth must become informed about the philosophy of their intended care provider. They also need to be prepared as to what is routine and "standard protocol" for the facility in which they intend to birth. The time to make these decisions is before the birthing day, not when you are in labour.

My focus for the past quarter century has been to bring relaxed natural birthing to the attention of birth professionals. I hoped that they would see and understand that all birth need not be approached with fearful anticipation and preparation, for sudden complication.

I am now placing my hopes on the most relevant players in this transformational and human experience—the birthing families.

Most parents hear only of "standard care" or "routine protocol or practice." These two phrases do not always mean that what the birthing mother will experience is only evidence-based treatment or that it is the best path to take. In their innocence and lack of information, parents approach their births with resigned submission. It's not that they don't care; it's that they don't know what they don't know.

Today I am optimistic that there will be a full shift in the direction of natural birthing that will show more sensitivity to the simple needs of the low-risk and no-risk majority of mothers who need little "standard" or "routine" care. I feel, though, that I will not see that happen in my lifetime.

I'm convinced now that this awakening has to occur first within the mind-set of the consumer families. They are not asking for more, or for special, treatment. They are asking for less. Parents are simply asking that if everything gives reasonable indication of normality, they be given the opportunity to birth calmly and gently as Nature intended, without drugs and other procedures intended to "give labour a jump-start" or "move it along."

It is they who are most transformed. It is they who must step up and accept the importance of educating themselves and actively seeking the birth professionals who will respect their work.

Hopefully, we will soon see that parents do not need to ask the same questions that families have been asking for the last 25 years. They won't feel the need to make a case for gentle treatment and kinder birthings. With education, they will recognise that they have the power to find and choose the care provider and the birthing environment that will make the difference in their lives and the lives of their babies.

The First HypnoBirthing Story

When I looked into my baby's eyes
for the first time, I knew at that moment
what real love actually is.

Maura Geddes

I left home at about 5:30 that January morning in 1990. As I slipped into my car, I felt the shock of the cold leather seats. The air was exceptionally cold and crisp, even for an early January morning in Concord, New Hampshire. Ordinarily, I would never venture out at that time of the morning in the peak of winter; but this was a very special day and time.

I knew there was no real rush, but I found myself hurrying out of my driveway and out onto the road to the city. The main road was deserted and dark, and it was mine for the taking. I was eager to reach Maura's house to learn how she was feeling, and to help her gather her things to bring to the hospital.

The city was quiet, but the still-prevalent holiday lights added to my excitement and feeling of celebration. This was the day that we had all been waiting nine long months for. It was finally here. The first HypnoBirthing baby was soon to arrive.

Just before I reached Maura's house, I had to slow down as I caught sight of a police cruiser neatly tucked away, with lights off, at the entrance of a local cemetery. I slowly drove past him, smiled, and rehearsed what I would say when he pulled me over on our way to the hospital after I had picked Maura up. I fully planned to fly past him and get his attention. I chuckled, picturing the drama of our arriving at the hospital with a police escort. Not! The cruiser was gone when we made that return trip around 7:30. Even in a perfectly scripted scene, I couldn't interject that drama into our first HypnoBirthing.

When I arrived at Maura's house, I found a perfectly relaxed woman, who had an obvious "ready-to-go" air about her. I was both pleased and relieved to see that she was in a light mood, smiling and conversant. We talked as she moved about, tidying and checking her house before we left. I saw no indication of fright or nervousness.

There were two friends who had also studied HypnoBirthing at the same time that Maura did. All three were expecting their babies around the same time, and I prayed that Maura would be the first to birth. I so wanted my grandbaby to be the first HypnoBirthing baby. I wondered how each of these three trusting pioneers would meet the start of labour. I also wondered how the hospital staff would meet their determination to have their babies naturally. Maura was the epitome of calm, and I knew that she was prepared. I was encouraged that the other two "first HypnoBirthers" would experience that same confidence.

When we arrived at the hospital, Maura was brought directly to triage and then admitted, even though the attending nurse found her to be in less than what is considered "active labour." Maura assured the nurse that she was experiencing regular surges. It was only then that Maura was told that her midwife was not available and that she would be attended by a midwife whom she didn't know. Once more I wondered how she would handle that bit of information. True to a very important affirmation in HypnoBirthing—"I will accept whatever turn my birthing takes"—the news did not stress or upset her.

She remained at that same level of opening for almost four hours. I know now that this is not uncommon for HypnoBirthing mums. Their labours very often do not conform to routine numbers on progress charts. Their bodies labour, but there is little change in their appearance. It is also not uncommon for them to very suddenly register a greater degree of opening in a much shorter time. Concerned that her labour was not progressing sufficiently to match the prescribed expectation, at about 10:30 in the morning her nurse suggested that she ". . . get up and get those muscles moving. It will speed up your labour." Maura was helped into a suggested squatting position, but with no preparation for squatting, she decided very quickly that she didn't care for the squat. She then began to walk, but got as far as the door, and said, "No thank you. I need to go back to relaxing now." She was tuned into her body and realised that the pace of her labour was stepping up. She needed to relax into her birthing body as she experienced active labour.

We heard little from Maura from that point on, except after she had listened to a woman in the next room scream steadily for a couple hours and beg for help from above. Maura opened her eyes and looked at me and asked, "Am I going to get to that stage?" The nurse answered, "Heavens no. You are way beyond that stage." Things were good.

Shortly after 1:00 P.M., Maura was completely opened and was advised to begin to forcefully push, while her midwife strenuously "stretched" her perineum, sometimes with both hands. Maura was obviously in pain through this episode, and called out to me to have the midwife stop tugging with her fingers. The midwife continued; and after some time, she performed an extensive episiotomy, saying, "This will help the baby come out faster." Thankfully, an episiotomy is seldom performed in most hospitals today. Birth attendants have learned that the folds of the perineum open by themselves and that the majority of cases call for patience to allow the natural expulsive reflex to move the baby down to crowning.

At 3:30 P.M. that afternoon, Kyle Patrick Geddes, the first Hypno-Birthing baby, was born. We were ecstatic. HypnoBirthing Baby #1 had arrived. We had no idea that there would be thousands—and even hundreds of thousands—to follow or that we would have representation in over 48 countries around the world. What a landmark day. We were simply happy in the knowledge that babies can come into the world with kindness, gentility, and respect for both mother and baby. Birth is, indeed, the greatest Celebration of Life.

We had gone full circle—from Maura, the first intended natural-birth baby in that county, to Kyle, the first HypnoBirthing baby. I can't even begin to express how moving this experience was for me.

Maura, without realising it at the time, had blazed a trail; and she did it without having the encouragement of many mothers before her who birthed naturally. Additionally, while her regular midwife encouraged her to have a natural birth, when it came time for her birthing, her midwife of choice was not there. I believe that on some deeper level Maura remembered her own birth and that allowed her to trust that her body, and her baby knew how to birth instinctively. The trail this woman blazed continues to widen today, for her footsteps have been followed by so many happy HypnoBirthing mums, who wanted gentle birthing but lacked a programme that would give them that choice.

We know that this is not the story of the first natural birth, nor was it the only natural birth. Women have been birthing naturally for centuries, but this was the first HypnoBirthing at a pivotal time. It proved that relaxed birthing that is free of stress and fear for all involved can be achieved routinely if the birthing mother is properly prepared and genuinely supported by her caring providers. It was significant at this time because some of the practices of Active Management of Labour, already with a foothold in other countries, were creeping into American births almost without notice. Hospital births were far from natural. Women who birthed in hospitals routinely expected to be medicated. In their apprehension, they demanded it. Today, we simply ask, is it not possible to acquiesce to the requests of the women who want less or none as it is to the women who demand more?

I chose to include this story not because it is the birth story of my daughter and grandbaby, but because it is a happy, positive birth story, and birth stories are important. Whether a birth story is a happy birth story or a not-so-happy birth story, it reveals the importance of parents taking the responsibility for knowing how they want to experience the arrival of their babies, whether their birthing takes place in a hospital, a birthing centre, or in a home.

This first HypnoBirthing mother, without the advantage of having watched many natural births on the Internet and in films and without the benefit of many happy birth stories, knew she wanted things to go differently; and they did. If this could happen for her, most certainly with the education, preparation, and choices that are available to you today, it could easily happen for you.

A Russian Mother's Comments about HypnoBirthing

*I recall it now, and I would say my
son's birth is one of the best moments in my life.
My doctor was shocked. She said she had never seen
anyone being so calm and relaxed during the labour.
My HypnoBirthing experience made me realise how wrong
our childhood attitudes are toward birth.*

Anastasia Ivanova, Moscow, Russia

Mongan Method of HypnoBirthing—Its Roots

I think I always knew and believed that birthing should be simple, instinctive, and even joyful for mothers, babies, and birth partners. I think I came here with that knowing, because from a very early age, I held a fascination for babies. I thought that babies should come onto this earth plane gently—in keeping with the beings that they are. I had heard people speak of babies as gifts from heaven, and I was thoroughly convinced that meant that babies are angels. Everywhere I looked; there was proof of it: Greeting cards at Christmas, pictures at church, comments from adults referring to a baby as "a little angel." For me, it all led to the same conclusion. Babies are angels.

As soon as I was old enough to make my wishes known to Santa, I asked for a "real baby doll." My pleas were heard, because I did receive a baby doll that was so nearly real that she could drink water and then expel the liquid instantly onto her diaper and her blankets. She was a little small, but so was I.

The following year when all my neighbourhood friends were asking for Shirley Temple dolls, I again asked for a baby doll; but this time I wanted a doll that was the size of a real baby. Once more, my wish came true; and I found a life-sized baby doll under the Christmas tree.

I didn't put her aside for weeks—her eyes closed when I laid her down, and they opened when I picked her up. She was perfect.

I wasn't much older when Mrs. Burrell, our next-door neighbor, brought her newly born baby home from the hospital. She very kindly tolerated my curiosity and let me spend time at her house just watching the baby sleep and watching Mrs. Burrell bathe her and care for her. The baby affirmed my belief. She looked exactly like the angels I had seen pictures of. I didn't even notice that she didn't have wings.

I was still very young—almost five—when I first heard a birth story. My mother and a group of her friends used to gather regularly at one home or another in the neighbourhood. They often brought their babies with them. I used to hide just outside the living room door when they met at our house. I would sit quietly and listen because sooner or later—mostly sooner—their conversation would focus on their babies.

One day one of the women talked about what she had experienced when she "delivered" her second baby. As I listened, I know that my jaw must have dropped to my chest. Everything that she was saying was not at all how I had pictured angels being born.

Her story was terrible. The entire story was punctuated with the words, "danger," "afraid," and "miserable." She told of her journey by ship from New York to California by way of the Panama Canal, just weeks before she was due to have her baby. She was afraid of water, but taking the longer boat trip was cheaper than going by train across the country. She was violently seasick from the very beginning of the trip, and it continued throughout the journey. Her doctor on the ship was afraid that her baby would not be able to tolerate the constant retching, and he was afraid that she would be thrown into labour prematurely. She was dangerously dehydrated and was experiencing terrible cramping. He was not at all encouraging about the danger she and her baby were facing if it continued.

When she arrived in California, she was taken to the hospital, "just in the nick of time." She continued to describe her labour that followed. This part of her story was even more frightening than what she had previously been telling the group.

She spoke of a long, hard, and horribly painful labour that led to foetal distress. The situation finally required forceps to pull the baby down through the birth canal. When she awakened from anaesthesia, she was informed that her baby had damaged her pelvic region so badly that it was unlikely that she would ever be able to have more children.

I couldn't believe what I was hearing. I felt sick. I asked myself why she would say those things. Angels are not born that way. God would never have let that happen. I ran to my room in tears.

I cried many more times over that story, and it wasn't the last time I was to hear it, because the woman who told the story was my mother, and I was the baby who damaged her body so badly.

I felt a tremendous guilt throughout my growing up years. My guilt eventually turned into resentment every time I heard the story. I hated the thought of it. It was all so wrong.

As I grew older, I began to really listen and hear the repeated messages of what I looked upon as the "war stories." Birth is scary and dangerous. The more I heard, the more I sensed that I was growing up in a family and a society of women whose thoughts were very much occupied with the trials of being a woman and the perils of giving birth. It almost seemed that every woman who had experienced birth felt somehow compelled and delighted to tell her birth story, and it was always bad and filled with anguish.

I remember very clearly the day my sister had her first menstrual period. It was as though my younger aunts were welcoming her into a sorority of female victims. They told me, "Your sister is a woman now. She has 'the curse.'" I really didn't know what they meant by "the curse," but I quickly caught on that being a woman and having "the curse" was a free pass to spending at least one day a month languishing emotionally and physically and being excused from any chores that were strenuous. This curse wasn't all that bad, I thought.

It would have been very easy for me, as a child, to get pulled into this abyss of victimisation—to succumb to the fear-filled discussion and become so fearful of birthing that I may have chosen to avoid birthing all together, as many women have done for many years. Or, I may have chosen to seek a surgical birth out of fear and a lack of good information.

I honestly think that my mother's birth story made me the strong advocate for instinctive and natural birthing that I am today. Instead of developing a fear of birth, I searched and developed a philosophy of birth. Her story served as a catalyst for me. It challenged me later to reflect on what I had been feeling all those years and ultimately to seek a more balanced, natural, reasonable, and logical view of birth.

In talking with birth advocates in recent years, I find that I am not alone in having been led to natural birthing because of a friend or family member who for years repeatedly told a horrific birth story to anyone who would listen. Others said that they, too, chose to become involved in natural birthing because of these kinds of stories and felt the need to try to change the view of birth for that same reason.

The real tipping point came when I was in high school. Our English class was assigned to write a research paper. This provided me with an immediate and high incentive to really dig into books on birth and to find what I was looking for. I chose as my topic "Achieving Safe and Gentle Childbirth." I thought it would be easy. I was so wrong.

I found mostly thick medical textbooks, so heavy that I could hardly carry more than one at a time. These books were also heavily laden with the discussion of dangers, risks, abnormalities, and cautions that doctors in training would likely encounter in their practices. In spite of the fact that only a small percentage of women presented with these abnormalities, especially back then, the books I found were solely devoted to "what ifs" and subsequent procedures to remediate the problems.

There is no arguing the point that this training and knowledge is essential and that these well-honed skills and techniques have saved the lives of many women and babies over the years. However, I was struck by the absence of discussion on normal birth. I was also amused when I read an interesting caution in one of the leading medical texts of the time. The book suggested that the physician should exercise caution when working with the educated, sophisticated woman who may harbour a notion that she knows how to bring a baby into the world. There it was—in print—an identified enemy of birth, rather than the giver of birth.

I felt that the absence of discussion on natural/normal birth left a serious void in obstetric education and could, over time, have influenced the manner in which some doctors interact with their birthing families. From everything I could find, I came away with the feeling that the people writing the books considered only the human body and not the emotional and spiritual human elements that accompany the person they will be working with, probably more intimately than any person other than a mate. There was no mention of the privilege doctors enjoy in being invited to assist at one of the most transformational events in a woman's lifetime.

It was, indeed, straight forward, didactic discourse with an obvious breach between the psyche and the soma. These writings shed light on a possible reason for why such a large number of doctors, even today, may seem so uncomfortable with requests for their support of families who present low-risk or no-risk, when the parents are looking for natural birth in a hospital setting.

Years later when I was living in Arizona, I was invited on three occasions to speak about HypnoBirthing before the OB/GYN club of a medical school. Each time, I asked the students, who were about to graduate in a few weeks, how many of them had witnessed a natural birth. I explained "natural" as opposed to "normal." Not one hand was raised. I explained further, and still not a single hand was raised. This, too, may explain why so many doctors are reluctant to give their support to natural birth. It's uncharted territory to them.

The most significant piece of writing that I stumbled upon came, not in the form of a medical text, but within the pages of an issue of *Life Magazine*. This particular issue came onto newsstands on January 30, 1950, the very time that I was gathering notes for my paper.

On the cover was a young mother holding her newborn baby. She was radiant and had a soft smile of satisfaction on her face. The title on the cover read, "Childbirth without Fear." Inside it read, "A Young Mother Gives Birth to Her Baby with No Fear, Little Pain."

It told of a programme at Grace New Haven Hospital in Connecticut that was adopting the theories of Grantly Dick-Read, an English obstetrician, who staunchly fought for acceptance and recognition of the proven fact that there is no need for severe, lingering pain in normal, uncomplicated birthing. That magazine and the Dick-Read book that I subsequently bought changed my life.

I knew I had found the "Grail." The book was quite philosophical, though not largely instructional or even methodical. I was ecstatic that I had finally found something that was in line with all the thoughts I had been clinging to for years. It even explained *why* it is that there doesn't need to be pain in birthing in the absence of special circum-stances. It was so simple and so scientifically logical—the Fight or Flight response within the Autonomic System. The logic was "hiding in plain sight." It showed me once more that normal birthing is more a philosophy and a belief than it is a technique or a method.

As I read *Childbirth Without Fear*, I was amazed to learn that Dick-Read had been putting these theories forward before medical boards and medical associations since the late 1920s and the early '30s. I found it hard to believe that he was silenced and grossly ridiculed. One paper after another that he forwarded was arbitrarily dismissed, with-out being read. When he persisted, his medical license was threatened.

Years later when I first became pregnant, I turned to that book and practically memorised every word. The main premise of the theory is that when the body is relaxed, the firing of neuropeptides in the brain are slowed, and, therefore, pain is lessened and often non-existent. The stress-free body is then able to function as it was created to function—without the self-defeating tension that can cause birthing muscles to shut down.

I fully accepted that fear is the enemy of the birthing room. I knew little of hypnosis at that time, and I didn't realise that self-hypnosis was what I was learning. I absorbed the logic like a sponge and relaxed daily. Soon I could bring myself into a deepened relaxed state within seconds. I faithfully carved out a portion of my life to relax every day. My body was so in sync with the whole idea. There was not a doubt in my mind.

I talked with my doctor and explained that I would be having the baby naturally. One must remember that this was at a time when all women were systematically anaesthetised during the birthing phase, and their babies were pulled out with forceps.

He smiled and agreed that he saw no harm in that. I truly don't think that he believed I was serious. Not being aware of how I was preparing for my birth, I think he merely humored me.

I laboured for a little under two hours in absolutely pain-free labour. My baby's descent was hardly noticeable to anyone but me—I did nothing to alert staff that my baby was moving to crowning. The baby easily moved down and crowned. I informed the staff that I was crowning, and then there was chaos. The doctor was not there. I was quickly transferred to a trolley and whisked down the hall to the delivery room. My legs were held together, and I was told to pant so that the baby wouldn't come out. The doctor still was not there.

In spite of my protestations that I wasn't supposed to have anaesthesia, my legs were strapped four feet into the air onto what looked like a series of rain gutters. My wrists were held with leather straps at the side of the table, my head was held, and the ether cone was forced onto my face. That was the last thing I remembered.

When I came out of anaesthesia, I was dreadfully sick and was told that I would see my baby in the morning, but I was not to mind the bruises on the side of his head from the forceps. I was upset, but said nothing to my doctor. I knew that I had had my natural labour, but felt cheated out of my completely natural birth. Just a couple more surges would have done it, but it would have to wait until "the next time."

The birth of my second son went the same sad way for all the same reasons. The labour was a little shorter and beautiful. But, once again, even though I reminded him of my intention for a natural birth, my doctor was not there; and he left no instructions for the nurses. They refused to allow me to simply let my baby be born. So as before, I awakened to an upset stomach and was sick most of the night. Again

I was told that I had a son and would be able to see him and hold him in the morning. I vowed, "Never again!"

When I became pregnant the third time, I promptly greeted my doctor on my first office visit with, "Dr. Massey, we've got to talk."

He looked at me and asked, "What do we have to talk about, Mickey? This is your third pregnancy. You know how it's done."

I smiled back and said, "Yes, but you don't. Twice you assured me that I could have my natural birth, and twice, I never saw you. I felt betrayed and let down. My babies were almost born when I was forced to take anaesthesia. I need to know that I can trust you to be there; to support me. If you don't feel comfortable doing that, I understand, but I'm going to have to walk." He repeated, "Walk?"

I continued, "I'll have to go somewhere else to find a doctor who will support me in this. I've lost two opportunities to have my natural birth, and I don't want to take a chance on losing another."

He paused for a moment, picked up his pen and began to write. He wrote down and recited all the things I had asked for. When he finished, he said, "There! Are you happy now?"

I spoke very quickly, and through a smile said, "I'm not finished. I also want my husband by my side in the labour room and the delivery room." To understand how outlandish this request was, you have to realise that in the late fifties, husbands were not allowed beyond the lobby of most hospitals. Most were sent home to wait for the call that would tell them, "It's all over."

He threw his pen down and said, "Oh, come on. You can't ask me to stick my neck out that far."

I again smiled and repeated. "I'm not asking you to go out on a limb. If you don't feel comfortable with this, I'll understand but I'll have to get another doctor."

He picked up his pen again and said, "Why not?" It was a very amiable conversation, and I knew that this time we were in sync. I could feel it.

He swore me to secrecy because we both knew that if word got out in that small town, the birth I was planning would never have occurred. My daughter was born in an hour and a half in the most beautiful birth that I could have imagined. My husband was not allowed to stay long after the birth, but I held her in my arms for more than an hour, and later walked down to the nursery to watch as they bathed her. Another first, since as mothers we were not allowed to be out of bed for a full day after giving birth. The next morning when they brought Maura to my room, the nurse commented that the whole hospital was talking about her birth and how fantastic it was. She then added, "But she's only 6 pounds, 3 ounces. I guess anyone could birth a baby that small without too much trouble."

My son Shawn was born two years later, weighing in at 8 pounds, 6 ounces, with only a little over an hour of labour and birth. There was no comment then about weight. His birth was as spectacular as Maura's was. I thought I had opened the door for all other women, at least in that community. My doctor's only comment was that he was amazed that anyone could endure that much pain without showing it. It was a very long time before there was another intentional natural birth in that hospital.

Soon the Lamaze Programme came into birthing rooms, and many of the births were natural (no drugs), if not altogether calm and relaxed. Women were awake, but often exhausted.

I believe that the Lamaze Programme could have worked and lingered, but many of the people who taught it felt obliged to lead discussions on how to cope with pain and moved away from the value of eliminating it.

Since women were no longer routinely anaesthetised, the concept of pushing the baby out came in, loudly and clearly. Many of the nursing staff, and doctors themselves, accustomed to seeing forceps as the major tool to bringing babies into the world, didn't believe that babies would come out their own.

I would cringe when I listened to women describe their births, but I found very quickly that women who have not experienced a calm and gentle birth were not too likely to applaud those who were doing it. I began to refrain from joining these conversations, knowing that few would believe me anyway. They didn't want to hear it. Surprisingly, that attitude sometimes exists today with both parents and birth professional alike.

It wasn't until years later when Maura became pregnant that the compulsion to set all of these thoughts down could no longer be ignored. The fervour began to build within me again. The teacher within me forced me to make up a small book for Maura and our two friends. With Maura's birth story and the success of the others, HypnoBirthing became an entity unto itself. The mission was well established.

In looking back on all of these years, I have to admit achieving the widespread acceptance that HypnoBirthing now enjoys has been an unbelievably steep uphill climb, mostly because of the reluctance of main-stream health care providers to acknowledge what is right before their eyes.

In making the journey, I've been fortunate in coming to know many very admirable birthing professionals—doctors and nurses and mid-wives, both Certified Nurse Midwives and Certified Professional Mid-wives—who are truly in birthing to serve the families they work with.

I look for the day when all birth attendants will become more sensitive to the emotional and spiritual human aspects of birth. I think that if doctors and other birthing staff would give natural birthing a chance, even for only a few births, they would also benefit from the relief and release of assisting at births that are joyful. As a licensed counsellor, I know how working with repeated war stories and human despair and disappointment can drain one's spirit. Doctors should be required to study instinctive birth, if for no reason other than the rejuvenation of their own spirit.

Thankfully, there are doctors and midwives and nurses—many of whom are now HypnoBirthing practitioners—who are able to see past that rigidity, and they view the mothers who are birthing as whole, healthy persons engaged in a wholesome, healthy human experience. These are the people who should be on the frontline of birthing, rather than practising joyful birthing one birthing at a time, as their patients request it.

Consumer families themselves are the answer to better birthing. We can only help them to be aware of the dream and to see themselves as the answer to achieving it. When that happens, most babies will enjoy the respectful, gentle, and calm birth of angels.

In HypnoBirthing you will be exposed to all sides of birthing so that you can make educated decisions. We don't make decisions for you. We do emphasise that it is important that no matter where you choose to birth, or with whom you choose to birth, just be sure that you feel confident that your decisions and your options are a good fit with your preferences about the manner in which your birth experience plays out.

The HypnoBirthing Philosophy

Just as a woman's heart knows how and when to pump her lungs to inhale, her hand to pull back from fire, so she knows when and how to give birth.

Virginia D'Orio

Our Mission Statement

The HypnoBirthing Mission Statement reflects an important part of our philosophy and purpose.

The administration, faculty, and teaching practitioners of the HypnoBirthing Institute are dedicated to providing birthing women and their partners a tried and proven method of birth education that guides and assists them as they prepare to experience birth in a peaceful and extraordinarily beautiful manner. It is a programme that considers the psychological and spiritual, as well as the physical, well-being of the mother, her birth partner, and the newborn infant, independent of context, whether that be in a home, a hospital, or a birth centre.

Mongan Method HypnoBirthing is built upon an educational framework of self-understanding, special breathing techniques, relaxation, visualisation, meditative practise, and attention to nutrition, positive body toning, and healthful family living. Most importantly, it fosters an air of mutual respect for the birthing family, as well as the health-care provider in a traditional health-care system or a complementary setting.

HypnoBirthing's philosophy and educational programme offers women an opportunity to explore birthing possibilities that are available to them and, in the absence of special circumstances, to step into a birthing experience that most nearly matches their birth vision.

The HypnoBirthing philosophy is based on the following premise:

- In the absence of a special medical circumstance, a woman's body should not be forced to do what it already knows how to do.

- Women's bodies and their babies know how to birth. The design is perfect and needs to be respected and unimpaired.

- Mothers and their babies should be treated according to the status of their own health, and not that of other women who may have special needs.

- Birth is a natural human experience. Each needlessly imposed procedure, test, exam, and interruption can upset the natural rhythm and flow and may cause the birthing to go askew.

- Each labour has its own time schedule. It may rest, or it may accelerate. The event should not be externally manipulated or managed if there is no special circumstance requiring it.

- Women's bodies are as sacrosanct during birthing as they are at any other time or in any other setting.

HypnoBirthing remains more a philosophy of the manner in which babies should be welcomed into the world than it is a "method" or technique for birthing. The basic tenet of the HypnoBirthing philosophy is that the birthing of your baby is a celebration of the most basic human experience of your lives. As such, birth and you, the family who is involved in this event, should be honoured and respected as the most relevant participants. The birthing should be experienced calmly, gently, joyfully, and peacefully, as well as comfortably.

When the suggestion to add "The Mongan Method" to the Hypno-Birthing title was first proposed, I fought it. I am convinced that when birthing families prepare for their own births with a conscious curiosity, they begin to understand the many medical and media myths surrounding birth. They educate themselves and they see these myths as just that—unfounded myths. They then approach the births as informed consumers.

The basic tenet of the programme is that childbirth is a normal, natural, and healthy human experience for the vast majority of women. When you are informed, you realise that when it comes time to birth your baby, the confidence that you develop in HypnoBirthing helps you to know that your birthing does not need to be accompanied by fear or severe pain and anguish. If you are healthy; if the baby you are carrying is healthy; and if you have had a healthy pregnancy, chances are in your favour that you will be able to anticipate and experience the labour of your choice, along with the other 90 to 95 percent of birthing women.

The HypnoBirthing view of birth is that it is a natural extension of the sexuality of a man and women; and, for that reason, we believe that birth is about them. It is about family fulfilment. It's about helping men to let go and free themselves from century-old programming that has eroded their role in birth and made them onlookers in one of the greatest and most important experiences of their lives.

It is about the manner in which they welcome a new little person in their family and into their lives, and it's about accepting responsibility for achieving the safest and most comfortable birth for their baby. Birth is not about science, although it is founded on science and supported by scientific evidence. More studies are supporting a natural approach to birth than ever before.

Families embracing the belief that birth is about them and the wonderful life-changing transition they are making into parenthood don't really need to be taught how to birth. They simply need to learn about birth. They come to understand that when the mind is free of stress and fear that cause the body to respond with pain, nature is free to process birth in the same well-designed manner that it does for all other normal physiological functions.

In spite of the fact that most births take place in hospitals, Hypno-Birthing does not believe birth is a medical incident. Healthy pregnant women are not diseased, nor are they ill.

The programme philosophy does not preclude the introduction of medical intervention, per se. It precludes the introduction of routine, arbitrary, unnecessary intervention.

Just as the animal mothers in Nature do not need a "medical lesson" to be able to bring their young into the world, human mothers also do not need extensive details of artificially fragmented stages of labour to instinctively bring their babies to birth. The bodies of healthy pregnant women instinctively know how to birth, just as their bodies instinctively know how to conceive and how to nurture the development of the babies they are carrying.

No matter how many children are born to a family, each child will experience birth only this once. He does not get a chance to do a retake. Emerging and just-born infants need to know that this is a place where respect, gentility, and love are practised. Especially at the beginning of life, they need to feel protected. In those first few moments of life, a baby can learn love, respect, and protection, or he can learn indifference.

The insidious growth of the second paradigm and the unexplainable blind acceptance of it by birthing parents tells me that no matter how many gains we make toward natural, instinctive birthing, it is not enough if there are still birthing experiences that are marked by indifference to the mother and baby's emotional and physical well-being. We have to somehow get the attention of those who, perhaps, don't even know that they are indifferent to what's right before their eyes.

HypnoBirthing guides mothers as they align with their own innate capacity to be able to give birth gently, comfortably, powerfully and joyfully. HypnoBirthing does not profess to offer preparation for births that are totally free of pain, discomfort, or unanticipated incidents. We do offer women an opportunity to explore the possibility of stepping into their birthing without fear or stress. Our experience over the past twenty-five years has allowed us to see these kinds of births repeatedly, and we've been sensitive to the way in which the couples leave their births touched with remarkable joy, fulfilment, and empowerment. We read it in their birth stories, and we hear it in their voices when they call or visit.

The HypnoBirthing philosophy will help you to learn to embrace your body's instinctual knowledge by relaxing into your birthing experience, and trusting in the many birthing gifts of nature that are already in place. You will want to let this experience unfold easily and gradually without interruption. You will gain confidence by rehearsing the birthing event. It is this confidence that will eliminate fear and fatigue and shorten your birthing time. The result of your preparation is a truly rewarding and satisfying birth that you and your partner and your baby are all a part of.

You will come to learn that women have been giving birth naturally and without intervention and instruments since the beginning of time. These are by no means new concepts. But the possibility of natural birth has been dismissed and even overridden for too many years. Even now, beliefs and the proof that support them are ignored by many.

In recent years women have been calling for their right to reclaim their birthing power. Women knew they had this capability from the beginning of time. It never occurred to the earliest of women that they didn't know how to birth. But through the years they have been taught to birth, and in such a manner that was actually contrary to their natural instinct. HypnoBirthing is helping women reclaim their ability to birth naturally.

Hippocrates and Aristotle were, perhaps, the first to extol a philosophy commending the efficacy of instinctive birthing. Birth was looked upon as a beautifully orchestrated natural human experience, designed to ensure the survival of the human race. There are many women who are clamouring for the return of gentle, instinctive birth, as evidenced by the many thousands of families who have sought natural birthing in the years since the inception of HypnoBirthing.

There have been many men in medicine down through the ages who have shared a philosophy of a simple and natural approach to birthing. These truly caring providers have supported birthing women and encouraged them to call upon their natural birthing instincts whenever possible. There are many doctors who have lent their respect and encouragement to birthing families when requested to do so.

One such doctor was Jonathan Dye of Buffalo, New York, who in 1891 wrote a book entitled *Easier Childbirth*. Dr. Dye pointed to the logic and scientifically back theory of natural birth when he wrote:

According to physiological law,
all natural, functions of the body are achieved
without peril or pain. Birth is a natural, normal
physiological function for normal, healthy women and
their healthy babies. It can, therefore, be inferred
that healthy women, carrying healthy babies,
can safely birth without peril or pain.

DR. JONATHAN DYE

More currently, Dr. Michel Odent, world-renowned advocate of gentle birthing, points out, "One cannot help a physiological process. The point is not to hinder it." He advises that birth attendants keep their hands in their pockets when they are by the side of a birthing mother so that the natural process can play out.

The late Dr. Gregory White, a supporter of natural birth, offers his view of the simplicity of birth in this excerpt from his book, *Emergency Childbirth*, a book written for the police and fire departments of Chicago.

"The most important thing for the lay assistant to know is that labour and the delivery of a child are normal functions, which Nature always tends to complete successfully.

"The women who deliver in taxicabs, ambulances, and police squad cars (or, unexpectedly at home) are usually those with short labours, and these are nearly always easy, normal deliveries. Since the babies in these circumstances are not suffering from the effect of anesthetics, or pain-relieving drugs given to the mother, they rarely require resuscitation.

"Generally speaking, mechanical assistance is rarely needed, but psychological or emotional support to the mother is almost always in order. This is usually given by means of a calm and confident manner and the frequent assurance that all is going well. Such moral support is given to the mother, not just because she is a fellow human being undergoing a trying experience—worthy as that reason is—but because calmness on her part and confidence in Nature, in herself, and in her attendant make it possible for her to do her part of the job better. Giving birth, at its best, is something a mother does, not merely something which happens to her (or is done to her).

"Reassurance and moral support are actually the major contribution of the attendant in most cases. This point should be stressed. (Complications) must be considered here (in the manual) because they sometimes occur in emergency childbirths. But they are rare—very rare. In over 95 percent of the cases of emergency childbirth, the emergency attendant will be overwhelmed with gratitude and widely praised as a hero or heroine, and he or she can smile at the knowledge that their simple task could have been performed by any bright eight year old."

When some people think of birthing, they associate it only with the physical aspect of its being the end of pregnancy and achieving the task of "getting baby out." While the baby's descent and emergence into the world are actually the end result of the physiological function of birthing, at HypnoBirthing we take a different and much broader view of this life-changing event.

We at HypnoBirthing see birth as deeply touching many facets of our human life, not just the physiological. With the birth of every baby, your personal life and responsibilities change.

The HypnoBirthing philosophy extends beyond birth into that adjustment period after birth. This is the time when you experience a phenomenal opportunity to assist your baby as he establishes a foundation of social and emotional responses that will last throughout his life.

As parents you will begin, if you haven't already, to assume the responsibility for seeing that your baby's womb life is calm, happy, and wholesome. His nutritional needs will become your nutritional needs; you'll become sensitive to his emotional needs, as well. You'll become sensitive to his need for safety, emotional well-being, and health. You'll also want to be sure that baby knows that he is welcome and that his actual reception into this world—birth—is equally as safe, calm, and gentle as possible.

This first birthday is also the most important birthday for your baby. How you look back on the birthing day experience is vital. It is said that there is no other single event that lingers longer in the mind of a woman than that of her birthing day. Deeper yet is the indelible imprint that the day of birth can leave in the mind of your baby.

It used to be thought that a baby is incapable of remembering events that occur when he is within the womb or at the time of his birth. Research conducted by the late Dr. David Chamberlain, author of

Babies Remember Birth, reveals quite a different story. According to Chamberlain, children, as well as adults, are able to recall, sometimes very vividly, the events of their lives within the womb, and they are able to act out events surrounding their births.

Preparing to welcome a baby is a life-changing experience, not just through pregnancy and birth, but long after. HypnoBirthing offers a remarkably simple, relaxed approach to this most important transition, as you step into your role as parent and become a family.

The philosophy is designed especially to serve the 95 percent of families whose pregnancies fall into the normal, low-risk, or no-risk categories. If you are part of this vast majority, HypnoBirthing will help you to experience this exciting time in your life with calm confidence as you look forward to your birthing day.

If, for some reason, your pregnancy and upcoming birth require special considerations, you will find that your HypnoBirthing techniques will beautifully complement whatever path your birthing will take, and it will help you remain calm, confident, and stress free. Additionally, the lessons you've learned in HypnoBirthing can help you to achieve a gentler, easier birth, regardless of any turn your birthing may take. Many women with special circumstances and even those who required surgical births have enjoyed happier and easier births as a result of their HypnoBirthing preparation. The gentle HypnoBirthing style also offered many benefits to mothers who had planned Vaginal Birth After Caesarean birthings.

If you have already embraced the concept of normal, natural birth as your choice, this book will provide an opportunity for you to explore its theories and learn more about how developing a calm approach to pregnancy and birth will enable you to prepare for a safer, easier, more comfortable and more joyful birthing.

Understanding the origin of many of the beliefs and myths surrounding birth that we, as a culture, have come to accept can assist you in making some of the decisions you will face in preparing for this most important time in your lives. This book will introduce you to ways in which you can connect with your pre-born baby and build a better understanding of your baby as a conscious little person, who is fully able to interact with you, even before birth. You can learn how to prepare your mind and your body in such a way that you will be able to achieve a happier birthing regardless of your present intent.

This book outlines the philosophy and many of the techniques used by HypnoBirthing families. You will gain much information and insight from reading this book. However, the comprehensive instruction and discussions covering specific methods, scripts, and demonstrations provided by your HypnoBirthing practitioner during classes, and even during your birthing, will prove to be invaluable.

The content of this programme is not intended to replace the advice and care of a birth professional. You should always seek the advice of a qualified professional caregiver for all pregnancy-related matters.

For information on HypnoBirthing classes in your area or for practitioner certification workshops, please visit our website at *www.HypnoBirthing.com*.

All natural birth has a purpose and a plan.
Who would think of tearing open the chrysalis as the
butterfly emerges? Who would break the shell and
pull the chick out prematurely? Who would force these
birth processes that are so perfectly designed?

Birthing Tips
I Learned from My Cat

Being an early teen and deeply involved with schoolwork, drum lessons, scouting, and cheerleading, my time and my mind were quite occupied. It would not be an exaggeration, however, to say that from time to time the Universe dumped situations upon me to keep me grounded as far as my quest for birthing information.

It happened on a beautiful late April afternoon in my twelfth year. I was in our backyard getting ready to plant sweet pea seeds. As I knelt over the bed I had prepared for the flowers, I felt a nudging at my hip. I turned and was surprised to see a very scrawny young tiger cat that looked much the worse for the wear of having been out on the streets. There were cuts on the edges of her ears and scratches on her face and head.

She continued to rub against me more emphatically. I saw this as a plea for food, so I picked her up and took her into the house to get some food. My mother took one look at my new friend, and shouted, "Where did you get that cat?" I explained and asked if I could keep it. Again, in a much elevated tone, my mother bellowed, "Get it out of here before it drops fleas all over everything." I took that as a "No" and quickly removed the cat, but I later sneaked food out to it. I did this for several days to make sure that the cat would stay. And she did.

The cat chose to cohabitate with chickens in a coop behind my grandmother's house next door. It was an unlikely pairing, but she had found a home. The cat and the chickens seemed mutually disinterested in each other. She settled into the coop and became one of the residents. I named her "Squatter."

I continued to sneak food to her, and eventually my mother gave in and said she could stay. I checked on her every morning. I was really never sure that she would be there when I went out to bring her food.

Shortly after, I realised that Squatter's weight gain was not entirely from the improved nutrition I was giving her. There was a small bulge in her tummy below her ribs. My grandmother gave a quick assessment. "That cat's going to have kittens." I was ecstatic. My cat was going to have kittens, and I would be her midwife.

There are several things that are worth noting about Squatter's choices in living style. She picked the very last nesting box at the far end of the coop where there was very little light. The box she chose was piled high with straw, as none of the chickens had used it. She seemed happy and looked like she was thriving.

I went out to feed Squatter one morning and noticed that something was different. Squatter usually slept curled up in a ball, but on this morning, she was lying flat on her side, with all four legs stretched forward. I knew she was in labour. I found a wooden milk crate and pulled it over to her nesting box. She was purring. I wanted her to know that I was there for her. I would be her midwife. I reached my hand out and patted her head and her neck. She abruptly shook her head and knocked my hand away. She settled in and began to purr again. I got the message. She wanted no interference. She let me know that she could do this herself without my assistance. I realised that I had interrupted her focus. She resumed a deep relaxation and continued to purr.

There was no change in Squatter's behaviour. She just lay there and purred. Soon I saw a ripple running along the side of her body. She remained still. The ripple finally reached her outlet, and a little head slipped easily out of her body. She raised her head to observe, and then leaned down to clean away the afterbirth. The little one crawled its way to the nipples, with Squatter just watching. Once the baby latched on, Squatter put her head back down and began to purr again. This first-time mum was in no way distressed. Her instincts were in full gear.

I sat there mentally saying "WOW! Yes! There it is. That's the way babies should be born." All that I had imagined—but with human mothers, of course—was there. I was witnessing it first-hand. What a beautiful gift I was given.

Soon there was another ripple that proceeded exactly as the first one had. There was still no change in Squatter's behaviour. She remained still and kept purring. Her second baby emerged as easily as the first had, and Squatter reacted in the same way. She had an almost cavalier manner about what she was experiencing. She began to clean this kitten.

Suddenly there was a raucous in the yard. Some dogs had come into the yard and were fighting. Squatter abruptly sat up. She paused and quickly took one of her kittens into her mouth, jumped out of her box, and disappeared through a hole in the back wall of the coop. I looked at the kitten that remained in the box and wondered, "What do I do now?" Squatter was gone, and I was left with a newborn kitten that kept crawling around the box, bobbing its head and looking for its mother.

I didn't need to worry for long. About fifteen minutes later, Squatter came running back through the hole in the coop, totally ignored me, and rescued her remaining kitten. I was relieved but also worried for the safety of Squatter and her family.

We didn't see Squatter for many days, but one morning my grand-mother called me to come to the chicken coop. There was Squatter in her nesting box and with four young kittens. Somewhere she had given birth to two more kittens. As I approached her and patted her, Squatter began to purr with pride and satisfaction. All was well in her world.

I thought for many long hours on that experience. It all made so much sense, but it also raised so many questions in my mind. Squat-ter's birthing reinforced many of my early convictions and gave me insights that were considerably broader than my simplistic rambling. "It shouldn't be that way." There was a comparison there that all women need to consider. The evidence that birth can be beautiful and simple may be a needlessly well-kept secret, but it's there. It's been there for decades, even longer, and its supporters have been voicing it.

The most important message to me was that Squatter was startled and afraid when the dogs came into the yard. Then she escaped. She instinctively shut down her labour and brought her babies to safety. Human birthing mothers aren't able to escape when they are afraid. Ironically, though, there are people who could effect a change in the level of fear that women experience as they approach their births. They are the caregivers who routinely witness birth as a joyful and calm experience. But who also choose to dismiss it when it is there, hiding in plain sight.

Hiding in Plain Sight

*. . .Theories are developed from
observations at the bedside of labouring
mothers, not in a laboratory.*

Grantly Dick-Read, M.D.

As I grew older, I searched for evidence that would support my premise that most births can be instinctive, physiological experiences if they are not needlessly managed and interrupted. I discovered that the biggest secret about birth is that there is NO SECRET. The truth that natural birth enthusiasts have been espousing for decades is clear and simple. My young cat Squatter knew instinctively what to look for when she prepared to birth; and when the time came, her body knew how to birth her babies.

Our animal mothers don't need to gather in groups and have explanations of why and how they should accomplish this natural function. No one teaches them the parts of their anatomy or the fractionalised stages of labour. More importantly, no one cheers them on to push their babies out.

There are many who would have us believe that the same rules of nature don't apply to human mothers. I once asked one of the medical students in my class how it is that animal mothers in nature can achieve quiet, peaceful births in a focused, relaxed state. The young man replied with stunning conviction. "The difference is that animal mothers are quadrupeds. Human mothers can't birth that way."

Parents today are becoming consciously aware that this kind of rationale will no longer suffice to quell sincere questions. Healthy, active, involved parents today are not content to listen while someone else describes their birth story and then directs the event in a manner so that it no longer is the birth story the parents envisioned. A healthy mother and a healthy baby are not the only things that matter in a birth summary. Parents want a birth that is fulfilling and respectful of the dignity of mother, baby, and the birthing experience.

Today's birthing family who is looking for a natural and calm birth is very much of the opinion that the manner in which the birth is handled definitely matters.

To this day, I reflect on those still "best-kept secrets" that my young cat knew. The message of Squatter's birth is blatantly clear—birth is simple, natural, normal, and healthy, if left undisturbed. It doesn't need to be manipulated, fixed, or managed.

The facts are obvious. The female body is created to conceive a baby; to nurture the development of that baby; and to birth the baby, gently and peacefully. The incomparable precision of the female reproductive system during pregnancy and birth, absent any unanticipated special circumstances, has been brilliantly provided by nature. And it is seen every day in many places.

It is absurd to think that we live in a world today in which so vast a number of families every day, with intent, give birth quietly, gently, calmly, and in comfort. At the same time, there are more women clamouring for these kinds of births for themselves and for their babies, and they are not being listened to or heard.

Every day many in the standard health care system see this happening; and, yet, they don't see it. Their eyes are open, but their minds are closed, and they choose to ignore it, marginalise it, and ultimately dismiss it; instead, opting to use procedures and protocols that are less beneficial, less gentle for both mother and baby, less effective, and less psychologically and emotionally sound.

It's been suggested that women be assessed to determine if they are possible candidates for postpartum depression. If the medical professionals who are well aware of gentle birth would open their hearts and minds and concern themselves with implementing birthing protocols that would make the birthing experience less traumatic, there would be far less need for remediating these conditions with pills.

HypnoBirthing mothers are so exuberant over their births that they feel they could take on any obstacle. If only someone would listen to their birth stories. The answer to avoiding birthing PTSD is hiding in plain sight.

The number of routine annoyances, interventions, and surgical births in some countries is rising to the point that it is out of control and will continue to reach astronomical levels until parents, the consumers of birth services, speak out and let their wishes be known. Birth professionals need to listen; to really see; and then consciously evaluate the birthing experiences that they attend. They need to consider the disparity between what parents are asking for and what they are receiving. Parents should not have to beg for what is readily evident. They should not have to resign themselves to the realisation that some doctors won't even discuss their requests. And so they end up in "resigned submission" doing what they say they don't want to do instead of seeking a different option.

A birth professional told me, "People who want those kinds of births should stay home." What? People who want to be treated kindly and with consideration and care can't get kindness and care in a hospital? Those were the words. Is that the message? Are they saying that if you want a normal birth, you don't belong in a hospital? Hospitals are only for people who don't care if they are not treated with kindness and care? Why are they indifferent and disinterested?

Parents need to be able to trust in their care providers, but in many metropolitan areas mothers don't even know the care provider who walks into the birth room to attend the birth. The results of the 2010 "Listening to Mothers" survey indicated that half of the responding birthing mothers met their care provider for the first time as he or she walked into their birthing room.

Decades ago, Dr. White, whom I quoted earlier in the HypnoBirthing philosophy section, was pointing out what he viewed was most needed in a routine, normal birth. Today, those same kind and encouraging words are still needed by the mother giving birth naturally and, even more so, by the mother who is experiencing a precarious birth and, perhaps, a bit of difficulty. If all birth attendants offered support, rather than brash words that exacerbate a mother's fear, births would progress so much faster. Care providers need to recognise that birth is much more than a physiological function. There is such an obvious need for providers to establish rapport and a mutual trust with birthing families. They need to step into their title.

The lack of rapport and wholesome communication is why birth is considered broken today. Ironically, it is being ignored by many of the very people who are at the heart of the dilemma—the parents themselves, the birth professionals whom the parents hire to attend their births, the attending staff at the facilities in which the parents choose to birth, and the general public. There has to be a change in thinking to bring this about.

Squatter's birth revealed some very important suggestions for how birthing mothers should be accommodated. The healthy mother who is seeking a natural, instinctive birthing is not asking more from those who provide her care, she is actually asking less. Here are some of the things a birthing mum may look for.

1. She needs to feel safe, secure, and comfortable. She wants to know that the people who are attending her birthing are kind and caring and respectful of her and the work she is doing. She needs to be free of unnecessary devices and apparatus that make her feel abnormal—raised bed rails that cage her in and wall out her partner, and machinery and equipment that is uncomfortable, cumbersome, and creates a sense of impending danger.

2. She knows it is not normal to have a needle or a heplock attached to her wrist so that she can remain hydrated. Her birth companion or doula is prepared to take care of her fluid intake and output.

3. She wants to be undisturbed in a quiet and calm environment so that she can focus on her birthing and connect with her baby as much as possible.

4. She would like her treatment to be kind, respectful, and caring, so that she can birth with dignity. She wants her care to be dispensed according to the status of her own health, and not on the basis of other birthing mothers' conditions.

5. She wants to be spared unnecessary comments that could cause needless apprehension and fear of what could come in later labour. She does not want to have her labour shut down out of fear.

6. She would like to be encouraged to adopt positions and activities based on her preferred comfort, unless doing so is not advisable for her. She enjoys the soft buoyancy of "nesting with pillows" to assist in relaxation.

7. She would like a minimum number of interruptions and would prefer them only when necessary or in the event of concern. Interruptions break the focus she has established and change the rhythm and flow of her labour.

8. She would like to be acknowledged as a responsible and aware person.

9. She wants to rely on her natural birthing instincts without prompts that may be contrary to the mindful programme that she is working with.

10. She wants to breathe her baby down through his descent and crowning with quiet prompts only from her birth companion. Her body, through the natural expulsive reflex, and her breathing will push for her. She wants to remain at ease without the stress of time constraints if the baby is tolerating labour well and shows no signs of distress. When the body is fully relaxed, advanced opening can occur gradually even when it appears to be sluggish.

11. She would like to be encouraged and accommodated in spending at least a whole hour or more in private, quiet family

bonding in the "afterglow" of the baby's birth to help baby adjust to the early period outside the womb. Visitors and staff should respect the need for baby to adjust to his surroundings and to the touch of only his immediate family.

Some families who are choosing natural, calm birth are welcomed into hospitals; many are welcomed into birth centres; some choose to birth in their own homes with a doctor in family practice or a certified midwife; some birth in birth centres. All women should have this opportunity, regardless of where they are birthing. But the facts are that some don't have any choices at all.

The people who are seeing this are to be commended for their concern and recognition of the need to do something about this horrific condition. But, along with this recognition, we need to see assessment of the birthing system. Why are so many mothers leaving their births overwhelmed with grief? They are mourning the loss of the vision they held for their birthing, because, in many cases, they have been denied their vision. Something must be done to make their birthing less traumatic.

Only when birth is looked upon as normal, and birthing mothers are looked upon as normal, whole beings, can one hope to have them leave their birthing beds feeling jubilant and anticipating their new role as a parent. Concern over a mother's post-natal mental health would be lessened.

If the medical system could just take a look at the faces and the stamina and attitude of mothers who are returning to natural, instinctive birthing, they would see an exuberance and spirit that nothing can parallel. HypnoBirthing mothers are so filled with joy and accomplishment over their births that they want to leave their birthing beds and shout it from the rooftops. We hear it in just those words all the time. It's not only the birthing mothers who feel fulfilled. Dads, too, tell us that the birthing experience has touched them so deeply in so many ways, and that they are closer as a couple then they have ever been.

A dad's eye view of birth that follows is typical of the birth stories we receive.

A Dad's-Eye View of Birth

Conny's water released at 5:30 A.M., but nothing else was happening. She told me to go to work. At 9 A.M., she said she was having surges, but nothing regular. I decided to come home, just in case. We pulled stuff together for the hospital and decided to go to my parents' house, since they live only ten minutes from the hospital.

By the time we got to their house, the surges had faded; and for the next few hours, Conny didn't have even one. She was getting a little worried because soon, it would be twelve hours from the time her water released; and if things didn't start, it could cause her to be induced at the hospital, which we didn't want.

After we ate, she lay down on the couch. We put on soft, instrumental music and started going through the relaxation scripts to put her at ease. Within ten minutes, she started having strong surges, five minutes apart. Within an hour, surges were about three to four minutes apart.

By the time we reached the hospital, Conny was having surges every two minutes. When she was assessed in the triage centre, she was already 7 to 8 centimeters open. She continued to do her slow balloon breathing through all of this, smiling and at ease in between the surges. It was unbelievable. It was just like we saw in the videos, but now it was so real.

We got into our birthing room at 6 P.M. The nurse set up the foetal monitor on her belly and then left us alone until Conny felt the need to start breathing the baby down. By 7:35 P.M., little Colin Emanuel Varga entered the world (only three and a half hours of labour)—no epidural, no episiotomy, no IV, no screaming baby, no pulling or pushing.

The doctor was absolutely fantastic. She was patient, understanding and encouraging, and used all the right terminology. Even the nursing staff was supportive. They were so surprised and impressed with this type of totally natural birth that we had a room full of nurses (between six to eight on a regular basis, and most of those were just there to watch). Everything went so well and so quick and so painlessly. As Conny put it: a lot of pressure, but no pain.

HypnoBirthing really works. We had such a wonderful experience, and Colin is alert, content, and happy. Best wishes to the rest of you, and Happy HypnoBirthing.

Mark & Conny & Colin, Canada

If only more birth professionals would look and listen to what is "hiding in plain sight."

From Celebration to Trepidation:
A History of Women and Birth

When one really thinks about the disparity between the way most animal mothers give birth and the way human mothers give birth, one cannot but wonder what happened. When mothers from other cultures are put into the mix, the questions become even more pressing. Where and why have human mothers in so many parts of the world abandoned their human instincts? What kind of strange quirk of nature brought this about? Why have women chosen to stray from nature? The answer—they had no choice.

The truth of the matter is that women today are just as capable as their counterparts in nature to call upon their natural birthing instincts, but those instincts have been blocked. **Women have been taught to birth.** They have been taught to birth in a way that is contrary to their very nature.

To truly understand the events that led up to our present-day thinking, where women birth the way they were taught to birth, we need to look back as far as 3000 B.C.

There is much evidence to support the belief that ancient women had their babies easily, with little discomfort or drama, unless, of course, there was complication. Historical records at the time of Jesus confirm that babies were regularly born in fewer than three hours. Hebrew women had their babies easily and comfortably within a short period of time. Naturally, of course.

Helen Wessels, founder of Appletree Ministries and author of *The Joy of Natural Childbirth: Natural Childbirth and the Christian Family,* offers us much research and study with Hebrew biblical scholars; and in her book, she emphatically says that there is no evidence to support the theory that women in ancient times considered childbirth a curse or that they suffered in childbirth. It was not uncommon for mothers to give birth away from their villages and unassisted. They then would return to their villages with their babies in their arms. We have only to look to the Nativity of Jesus to read of such a birth.

In other parts of the world—Spain, France, the British Isles, and old Europe—the lives of the people centred around their gods of Nature and motherhood. They honoured Mother Nature, Mother Earth, and their top deity, Mother Creator. Because women were able to naturally bring forth children, they were revered and considered to be connected to Mother Creator. Pictures of statues found in their ancient stone temples depicted women, fully rounded in pregnancy and with full breasts. Some statues even show a baby crowning or emerging from the vaginal outlet of their mothers.

These primal people regarded birth as the highest manifestation of nature. Ceremonies centring around the happy occasion of birthing were of high importance. When a woman was to give birth, people of the village would gather around the pregnant mother praying to their gods that the child would be healthy, wise, and strong. Birth was a holy rite and a "Celebration of Life." There was nothing that suggested that labour was the long, dreadful, and painful ordeal that it later was believed to be.

Women were nurturers and healers, developing herbal brews and administering healing medicines. All healing came at the hands of the healing spirit in women. They collaborated and exchanged learning, overseen by the wise women of the village. Men were the gatherers of the herbs, food, and building materials. Their roles were different, yet equal in their society.

Eventually, men took the lead in medicine. Even then, there was no change in attitude or approach to birth.

Both Hippocrates and Aristotle, leaders of the Grecian School of Medicine, were sensitive to the emotional and spiritual needs of women who were birthing. They both wrote that a woman's needs and her feelings should be accommodated during childbirth. Neither wrote anything about danger or pain and suffering in his notes. Are we to believe that the presence of pain in normal birth was not recognised and simply went unnoticed? I think not.

Hippocrates believed that birth is a natural experience and ". . . should not be interrupted with 'meddlesome interference.'" He established midwifery for the purpose of giving birthing women emotional support. He also believed that in birthing, Nature is the best physician.

In his notes, Aristotle wrote of the mind and body connection and emphasised the importance of deep relaxation during birthing to relieve any discomfort. In the event of a complication, he also recommended relaxation so that the complication could be treated and resolved.

They both advocated for a support person to be with a birthing woman (today's doula), and Hippocrates was the first to organise and present formal instruction for midwives. With this distinction, many other women moved more openly into the realm of healers. They regularly tended to the ill of the villages with their brews and tinctures.

During the last century before the birth of Jesus, another leader from the Grecian School, Soranus, a medical student, put the writings of Aristotle and Hippocrates into book form. Soranus emphasised the importance of listening to the needs and feelings of women who are giving birth. He also advocated using the power of the mind to achieve relaxation in order to bring about an easy birth. Like his predecessors, Soranus, too, made no mention of pain, except when he wrote about complicated, abnormal birth. If there were no complications, under the watchful eyes of Soranus, women were kindly and gently cared for in a normal birth. This attitude remained for several hundreds of years.

At the end of the second century, a new wave of political governance, strongly influenced by the church hierarchy in Rome, began to sweep through all of Europe, bringing with it decrees of contempt for anything related to the worship of nature. Their goal of abolishing all rites and ceremonies previously practised in honour of nature was carried out swiftly and completely. Birthing rites and ceremonies were forbidden by the new laws, and the iconic statues and stone temples were destroyed.

Because women were living symbols of the connection of women to a "Mother Creator," it was essential that they be controlled and restrained. Since only God could heal, the talents of the wise healers were discredited and used as proof that they drew their power from the devil. Witchcraft, a very honoured position within the early villages, was forbidden by law. They could no longer go out to tend to the ill and were forbidden to be with birthing mothers. Pregnant women were segregated and confined to their homes. But for the healers, midwives, and doulas who were at the core of the strong female presence, the price to pay was much higher. For them, the punishment was death, usually by public burning at a pyre in the centre of the village square.

The condemnation of women escalated as the authority for all medical practice lay in the hands of the local priests and monks. More laws decreed that doctors could minister only to those who were "deserving ill" and only then after seeking permission. Women were accused of being seductresses; and, therefore, the unborn babies they were carrying were conceived, not through a connection with a Holy Mother, but rather through a connection with the devil. Because they had conceived their babies in "carnal sin," were undeserving and were totally isolated during their births. Under fear of execution, no one could accompany a birthing mother. Doctors were forbidden to assist, even in the case of a complication.

The fervour of the war against women became so heated that at one point in time, a council meeting was called with the intent of declaring that women were not even human beings.

With midwifery having been abolished, the only person who could attend to a woman in the event of a complication was the goat gelder, who swiftly cut the baby from the mother, and she was left to die. The life and soul of her baby was considered saved, and therefore the incident was justified.

It was at this time that what was known as "The Curse of Eve" was embedded into the translations of the Bible by Clement, who was later sainted. Previously there had been no mention of a curse. Other church leaders became blatant in their dismissal of the treatment of women.

---

* Pope John Paul II many times during his long papacy, in letters and in speeches, offered an unprecedented public apology, asking for the forgiveness of the world for the sins of those acting in the name of the Catholic Church for the attacks upon Jews, women and minorities, victims of the Spanish Inquisition, Muslims killed during the Crusades, and other infractions. He cited the burning at the stake of woman, and the violation of women's rights, and other Church abuses over the past 2,000 years. ("Pope John Paul II." Wikipedia: The Free Encyclopedia. Wikimedia Foundation, Inc. August 17, 2015. Web. August 21, 2015. <*https://en.wikipedia.org/wiki/Pope_John_Paul_II*>).

In the years between the 2nd century and the 16th century, matters became much worse for women and birthing. Later other church leaders became blatantly dismissive of what was happening to women. One such leader in Germany was quoted as having said, ". . .if a woman suffers and dies in childbirth, so be it. That is what she is there for." Midwives who attended birthing women were called *Wehmutters* or "mothers of woe." It was still generally considered that birth was painful and dangerous.

In the 15th century, the lost books of Soranus were discovered, and the world began to take notice. The madness and chaos of the former period had subsided. The Reformation caused the Roman Church to examine many aspects of its policies, doctrines, decrees, and practises. Much was changed. The blatant mistreatment and executions of women were lessened; however, they were not entirely out from under the veil of abuse and subjugation. It was even worse for women who were not of higher social standing. The poorer women were shown no mercy.

In 1853 and 1857 when Queen Victoria of England insisted on having anaesthesia for her births, its use in obstetrics became firmly established and was widely used routinely. It became the choice of doctors for achieving the obstetrical goal of "getting baby out." Because it was too cumbersome to administer anaesthesia in a home setting, upper class mothers and their babies made their way into hospitals. Lower class women remained in the care of midwives.

In the mid-1900s, following the lead of Dr. Joseph DeLee, doctors began to view all births as problematic. It was decided that since normal births were rare in hospitals, interventions should be applied to all births to prevent the evils of labour. These preventions included all interventions utilised in modern obstetrics for highly complicated cases.

. At about the same time, the English obstetrician Grantly Dick-Read introduced his theory that pain was not an inherent part of birthing. Based on his experience, as he said, ". . . at the bedside of birthing women," he forwarded what he called the Fear–Tension–Pain Syndrome, emphasising that when a mother is taut, her body is also taut. Dick-Read's papers were not accepted, and he became the object of ridicule.

Also in the mid-1900s, Dr. Fernand Lamaze brought into the birthing scene the first real approach to natural birthing that took hold. Dr. Lamaze advocated unmedicated, natural births. Women were to remain awake and use their power of focus and breathing to distract them from the pain of labour. It was then that women were taught how to birth. They learned that they were to push their babies to crowning.

After Dick-Read, one doctor—Robert Bradley—looked upon Grantly Dick-Read as a hero and patterned his birthing programme with relaxation, as recommended by Dick-Read.

When we look back upon these events with our modern knowledge, we understand more clearly how fear of complication and resulting death, not fear of birthing, caused women to look upon labour with horror. Extreme fear created extreme tension, and the tension, in turn, resulted in a taut cervix, unable to perform its natural function. Those who lived through the ordeal, as well as those who witnessed it, attested to the agony that was experienced in birthing.

Birth was still very low on the list of priorities among medical people. Maternity wards were filthy and staffed primarily with physicians who were inept or alcoholics.

As a result large numbers of women were dying, not from childbirth but from "child-bed fever." The remnants of this period have contributed enormously to a fear of dying in childbirth. Obviously, this is a fear that is no longer valid today. It wasn't until Florence Nightingale used her clout as an exemplary fundraiser that the maternity wards were cleaned up and the professional level of staff was improved.

The stories and the scripts were firmly set. Birth, once a major celebration, had been turned into something that was filled with dread and trepidation.

It is not difficult to understand why women to this day feel so much anxiety over the thought of birthing. However, as we understand the cause, we must also understand and realise that hundreds of years have passed since that bleak period of time in birthing history. We also can understand that there is no longer the need for women to harbour a dread of labour. These thoughts are no longer valid in today's birth settings.

Today's women have many choices in birthing. They have many opportunities to explore those choices. The first and most important choice being the selection of a childbirth preparation programme that will help them to seek, explore, and find the people and the environment that feels "right" to them.

HypnoBirthing's philosophy and educational programme gives women the opportunity to explore their choices; and in doing so they are able to create the possibility of stepping into the birth that they feel is a right fit for them. They can decide whether or not what has become routine for other women must be a part of their birthing. They can learn, look at what currently exists, and choose "What can be." That is their prerogative as they fulfill the single life human function that is theirs alone to experience.

Today, even with evidence to the contrary, an incredible number of people in maternal services, and even women themselves, continue to accept the myth that pain and problems are an inevitable part of birthing, and that birthing has to be a laborious ordeal that leaves both mother and baby exhausted. It is widely thought, even by the birthing mothers, that the best thing they can do for themselves is to turn the birth experience over to their care provider and attending staff and depend upon them to guide them through the experience. Why do these myths persist? Why do women's bodies, perfectly created to birth, shut down even before they start labour? Why do so many women require that their babies be extracted surgically—a procedure that forty years ago was so infrequent that it was regarded with surprise?

The answer can be found in one word: fear.

How Fear Affects Labour

To those who say it is just not possible to
birth naturally and without pain, I say,
"But what if we're right? Wouldn't it be wonderful?"

Lorne R. Campbell Sr., M.D.

I once met a vivacious young woman who was five months pregnant. She glowed as she talked about her pregnancy and how she had felt so wonderfully healthy. She spoke of all the things she was doing to prepare her body for birth—swimming, yoga, walking. In the middle of all of this happy conversation, she paused, clenched her fists, and said, "But I can't even think about THAT day. I have totally blocked out all thought about the birth. I can't bear the thought of what it will be like. I am so scared."

"Terrified" is the more appropriate word to describe what women are feeling as they approach what should be among the most exciting moments of their lives. This young woman, obviously very sophisticated and very much in control of the events of her life, took on an air of helplessness when it came to the thought of birthing. Sadly, she represents women in many parts of the world. It is a travesty that manufactured fear, leading to manufactured consent, casts such a cloud over the otherwise joyful excitement that couples should feel as they anticipate becoming parents.

The belief in pain surrounding childbirth is so strong that instead of questioning the validity of the concept, there have been many efforts to rationalise its importance and to attach some reason and higher purpose to it.

Some programmes teach methods that attempt to take your focus away from pain so that you will not be so aware of it. Others will tell you that pain is a very important signaling mechanism, a sort of biofeedback that alerts you to where you are in your labour. The theory is that if you can identify the degree of severity and the frequency of it, you will be better able to determine where you are in labour and what coping techniques you will employ to continue. Still others suggest that you look upon it as an unavoidable but useful friend that can be tolerated, worked with, and learned from. There are even those who revere pain in birthing and see it as a vehicle through which to achieve the empowerment of womanhood. It has been suggested that we learn to honour pain, as other societies do, for the strength it builds in our character.

These programmes feel that because pain has to serve some purpose, it must be rationalised and accommodated in some way. For most women, these are not convincing arguments. Pain is still a four-letter word. Accepting the belief that it is necessary creates the very situation they want to avoid.

For those who refuse to examine the theory that there is no physiological reason for pain in birthing, the way to accommodate it is to provide a plethora of drugs that the birthing mother can escape into. For the pregnant mothers looking forward to such relief, the drugs are offered, not as a last resort during labour, but rather as a menu, presented within the childbirth education class so that selections and decisions can be made early on. These mothers want to believe that the drugs won't cross the placenta and affect their babies. No one tells them that the placenta has no barrier. And so they go into their labours believing that their birthing bodies are inadequate, but they can be "delivered" by drugs and technology, even when these interventions take them further away from normal and gentle birth for their babies.

Occasionally one of the women in a HypnoBirthing class will ask, "Why don't we human beings have our babies the way cats and dogs and horses and other animals do? There's nothing wrong with their labours." My reply is always the same: "Yes, why don't we?"

Medical professionals have long stood by the argument that pain is considered the "watchdog of medicine." Pain, they tell us, sends a signal that something is wrong. If that is true, we must make an exception for all other mammals for which labour is a natural, normal function.

We know that horses and other "dumb" animals will delay the start of their labours or shut them down when they don't feel comfortable with their environment or they feel endangered—just as my cat Squatter shut down her labour when she was in fear of the dogs nearby. Is it not unreasonable to think that women's bodies have that same instinctual capacity? Why do we believe this of animal mothers, yet refuse to consider it for human mothers?

I am frequently asked to prove that HypnoBirthing works—that eliminating fear and other stressors and building trust in the birthing process results in a truly safe, healthy, happy-baby and happy-mother outcome. This, in my mind, is like asking me to take a finely tuned, precision instrument that has been broken and prove that it would work perfectly had it not been broken in the first place.

The concept of birth has been distorted. The spirit of women with respect to their innate birthing power has been broken. We can do nothing about the millions of broken births that have already taken place, but by seriously looking at the effect of fear—the powerful emotion that clouds our thinking and causes the birthing body to break down and deviate from its natural course—perhaps we can keep the finely tuned, precision bodies of women whole for future generations.

Your Marvelous Birthing Device: The Uterus

Your uterus is perfectly designed to assist you to birth your baby. When we understand the way in which the uterus functions naturally when unencumbered by fear, the concept of easier, more-comfortable childbirth immediately becomes obvious and, therefore, attainable. This very brief explanation and the illustrations are, indeed, the crux of our entire programme. It is exactly this process of your body that you will work with during labour. This is the way the birthing muscles are designed to work—in perfect harmony.

There are three layers of muscle in the uterus. The two layers with which we will be concerned are the outer layer, with muscles that are vertical (aligned up and down with your baby), and the inner layer, with muscles that are horizontally circular (surrounding the baby).

The circular muscles of the inner layer are found in the lower portion of the uterus. As the illustrations show, the circular muscles are thickest just above the opening, or neck, of the uterus, called the cervix. In order for the outlet of the uterus to open and permit the baby to easily move down, through, and out of the uterus into the birth path, these lower, thicker muscles have to relax and thin.

The Uterine Layers

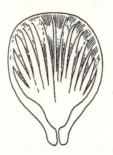

The outer longitudinal muscle fibres of the uterus

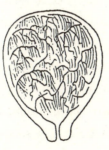

The middle muscle layers, interwoven with blood vessels

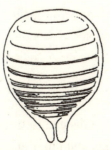

The inner circular muscle layers found mostly at the lower part of the uterus

The stronger muscles of the outer layer of the uterus are vertical fibres, with a stronger concentration at the top. They go up the back and over the top of the uterus. As these muscles tighten and draw up the relaxed circular muscles at the neck of the uterus, they cause the edges of the cervix to progressively thin and open. In an almost wave-like motion, the long muscle bands shorten and flex to nudge the baby down, through, and ultimately out of the uterus. It is this tightening motion that many HypnoBirthing mothers report as being the only sensation that they experience during the thinning and opening phase of labour.

When the labouring mother is in a comfortable state of relaxation, the two sets of muscles work in harmony as they were intended. The surge of the vertical muscles draws up, flexes, and expels; the circular muscles relax and draw back to allow this to happen. The cervix thins and opens. Birthing occurs smoothly and easily.

The Surge Breathing technique that you will learn and practise in your classes is designed to help you to work in concert with these birthing muscles. Combined with the relaxation practice you will do on a daily basis at home, this will help you learn to bring your body into a relaxed state that can make your surges more effective and substantially shorten your labour. You will learn to visualise the lower circular muscles as soft, blue satin ribbons, flexible and totally nonresistant to the draw of the upper muscles.

Fear: The Enemy of the Birthing Room

We have seen how the birthing muscles are beautifully orchestrated to work. Now let's look at what happens when the birthing mum is tense and fearful.

The effect of fear upon labour is not subtle, insidious, or complex. We see it in front of us in every uncomplicated birth with every labour that is slow to start or delayed or that later slows or rests. Yet this obvious emotion, one of the strongest and most debilitating that we know, is basically ignored. Instead of being helped to recognise the harmful effects of fear upon the body, mothers are asked to surrender themselves to drugs, technology, and manipulation to force their bodies to do what they are naturally capable of doing when left to their own means and when the circumstances are "right" for birthing.

The negative physical effect of fear on labour can be traced to the function of the body's Autonomic Nervous System (ANS). The ANS is the communication network within our bodies. Its main function is to interpret messages it receives, determine what action should be taken as a result of the message, and then immediately communicate that directive to the other systems of the body. The responses to impulses that are transmitted through the ANS are not subject to our conscious control and are, therefore, involuntary.

For the purpose of looking at the impact of stress upon birthing, as well as the beneficial effect of calm, we'll need to look at the two subsidiary systems within the ANS—the Sympathetic System and the Parasympathetic System. These systems control those responses that cause us to accelerate or slow our breathing, to blink our eyes, to step up or reduce our heartbeat, to arrest or maintain our digestive processes, and to carry out many other functions of the body.

The Sympathetic System is triggered when we are stressed, frightened, or startled. Therefore, I call this part of the system the "Emergency Room." It is the role of the Sympathetic System to act as the body's defence mechanism. It instantly creates the "fight, flight, or freeze" response within the body. When it is in motion, it causes the pupils in the eye to dilate, increases the speed and the force of the heart rate, and causes the body to startle and move defensively. It suspends activities such as digestion. Most importantly, it closes arteries going to organs that are not essential for defence. It prepares the body to deal with emergencies and danger. It is designed to save your life.

The activities of the Emergency Room put you into a state of alert. For that reason, you should be spending no more than 2 to 5 percent of your life in the Emergency Room. It is like a "rainy day fund," and it shouldn't be tapped into on a regular basis.

On the other hand, the Parasympathetic System, which I call the "Healing Room," keeps the body and mind in a state of harmony and balance. It maintains the body functioning in a state of calm, slowing the heart rate, reducing stimulation, slowing the firing of harmful neuropeptides, and, in general, keeping us in a state of well-being. The Healing Room restores and maintains the normal functions of our bodies. We should be living 95 to 98 percent of our lives in the Healing Room.

How does this relate to birthing? The Sympathetic part of the nervous system responds not just to actual threats, but to perceived threats. The mother does not need to meet the saber-tooth tiger face to face in order to feel fear. In other words, the negative messages that a mother constantly receives are processed as being real. Over time, these negative messages become part of her belief system and compromise her body's chemical balance on a regular basis. They affect her emotional state and that of her pre-born baby.

When the mother approaches labour with unresolved fear and stress, her body is already on the defensive, and the stressor hormone catecholamine is triggered. Her body is sent into the "fight, flight, or freeze" response. It is believed that catecholamine is secreted in large amounts prior to and during labour.

When circumstances are such that neither "fight" nor "flight" are appropriate, as in the case of labour, the body naturally chooses the third option: "freeze." Since the uterus has never been designated as part of the defence mechanism of the body, blood is directed away from it to the parts of the body involved in defence. This causes the arteries going to the uterus to tense and constrict, restricting the flow of blood and oxygen. Labour and birthing nurses and midwives have told me of seeing uteruses of frightened birthing women that are white from lack of blood, just as a person who is experiencing extreme fright often has the blood drain from his face.

With limited oxygen and blood, vital to the functioning of the muscles in the uterus, the lower circular fibres at the neck of the uterus tighten and constrict, instead of relaxing and opening as they should. The upper vertical muscles continue to attempt to draw the circular muscles up and back, but the lower muscles are resistant. The cervix remains taut and closed.

When these two sets of muscles work against each other, it causes considerable pain for the labouring mother. The situation can also have an adverse effect on the baby. The upper muscles push to expel, forcing the baby's head against the tightly closed lower muscles that refuse to budge. In addition to the pain that this causes for both mother and baby, labour can be drawn out, or it can even shut down. Thus, we hear from mothers whose labours end in a surgical birth lament, "I was told my uterus wouldn't open." Limited oxygen in the uterus also means that the supply of oxygen to the baby is compromised. Over a period of time, this can be a cause for concern. The situation often is labeled "failure to progress" (FTP), and it usually results in intervention. It is interesting to note that the very same initials, FTP, are used to abbreviate both Grantly Dick-Read's Fear–Tension–Pain Syndrome and the failure to progress that it causes. What labour needs is not more urgency or prompting to "move things along," but more awareness of the importance of calm, relaxation, gentle encouragement, and assurance that actually can move the labour along faster.

Regrettably, Dick-Read did not live long enough to see his theory buttressed with the discovery of endorphins. Still more regrettable is that, even with this knowledge in hand today, few medical caregivers are opening their minds to the relationship that exists between the birthing experience and the ANS, with its ability to secrete endorphins, the "feel-good" hormones that relax the muscles and allow the body to open, as well as the stressor hormone catecholamine.

Attempts to speed the birth of a baby only result in more pain for the mother and the baby, and frustration on the part of caregivers, as the baby's head pushes against muscles not yet relaxed and open enough to accommodate it. HypnoBirthing allows for the body to work at its own pace and facilitates easier birthing by using relaxation and visualisation to speed the release of endorphins and effect an even shorter labour.

You and your birthing companion will be taught how to identify emotional stress before and during labour and how to release it. You will learn how to bring yourself into a deepened relaxation. When you are free of fear, you can achieve a relaxed state from the very onset of labour. Verbal and physical cues that you and your partner have practised will help you to maintain a state of calm from the very start, as constricting hormones are overridden by your body's natural relaxants.

Learning to understand the benefits of living in the Healing Room— and avoiding people and situations that place you in the Emergency Room—is a skill that will infuse calm into your everyday life. It will greatly enhance your relationship as a family, as well as ensure a calm and gentle birth.

Releasing Fear

Preparing women for birthing by educating them in the true physiology of their birthing muscles, and the need for the mother to be free of tension, was the backbone of Dick-Read's work. This concept appealed to the intellect of many women in the middle of the last century, and it was enough to inspire them to break with traditional attitudes and bring their children into the world unmedicated and alert.

Free of debilitating fear, those who subscribed to the philosophy of natural birth were free of anaesthesia, free of needless management of their birth, and, for the most part, free of the discomfort of labour.

Most births were attended by family doctors, a person who was known to the birthing mother probably from the time that she, herself, was a child. There was a long-standing trust established in the doctor/mother relationship. Mothers did not expect labour to be a picnic, but their labours were not anticipated with the fear that exists today. Birth, actually, was rather simple. Standard birth consisted of mothers, who with a little Demerol were able to bring their babies to crowning with little fuss. At that time, they were totally anaesthetised in time for the doctor to arrive to extract their babies with the help of forceps.

If you are like most pregnant women, you will find that as you move through these days and months of pregnancy, you will be met with a whole new set of feelings, anxieties, doubts, questions, decisions, and tasks that you never had to consider before. Some of these will centre on your pregnancy, labour, and birthing; but there may be more that will cause you to look at the many transformational experiences that bringing a baby into your life will present. This is natural. As you prepare your mind and body for your baby's birth, you will want to be ready in this regard also—free of any fears, reservations, or limiting thoughts.

It's helpful for both you and your partner to be able to identify feelings, experiences, or recollections that may be painful or hurtful, thus limiting your ability to approach birthing free of harmful emotions. Take a look at those emotions that may foster a feeling of uneasiness, meet them head-on, and release any conflict you may be harbouring (consciously or subconsciously) because of them. Once you have been able to work through and resolve lingering emotions, limiting thoughts, experiences, or memories that could stand in the way of an easy birthing, you will have a better sense of your own ability to approach the birth of your baby with trust and confidence.

Thoroughly search your inner feelings to discover the areas that you feel very confident about and those that you need to work through so that you can resolve any fears or misgivings that you are holding. Brushing aside matters that concern you may help you to get through your pregnancy, but these concerns can easily surface as fears when you are in labour, and they can affect the course of your labour. You will want to take advantage of the opportunity to talk with your partner, your birthing companion, or a good friend who can help you explore and discuss any thoughts that could be troubling you.

Your HypnoBirthing practitioner will help you inventory and identify those areas of your life that could possibly serve as obstacles. The practitioner will help you work with fear-release sessions in class. If you still feel you need some assistance in releasing lingering fears after you do the sessions in class and talk with your partner and friends, ask your practitioner for a private session. If you are not able to work with a trained practitioner, you may find it helpful to seek the counsel of a hypnotherapist to do release work with you. A fear-release hypnotherapy session is truly one of the most effective ways of eliminating toxic emotions.

Listed below are just a few areas of concern to pregnant women that surfaced in the early nineties as a result of Dr. Louis Mehl-Madronna's study on turning breech babies with hypnosis. Your own inventory may reveal other issues that you would like to resolve.

- **Your own birth**—What stories have you heard about your own birth? Are they positive and encouraging, or negative and frightening? Do you feel that you will duplicate your mother's labour? If what you've been told is less than encouraging, you might want to work on establishing that you are not your mother, and this is not her pregnancy. You are an entirely different person at a different time and under different circumstances and are preparing for your birth differently.

- **Others' birth stories**—Have you been surrounded with stories of joyful birthing, or have family members impressed upon you "family patterns" of long labours, back labour, severe pain, and medical intervention? Again, you do not need to assume the experiences of the people who are relating these stories. There is no reason to believe that you will birth as they did. Work at checking those kinds of thoughts so that you don't bring their past baggage into your birthing.

- **Previous labours**—Has your own experience with labour been easy and satisfying, or are you carrying recollections of an arduous ordeal? If you had a less-than-satisfying labour, take hope in the fact that you are better prepared for an easier birth this time, and you now can approach birthing with more knowledge and planning than you did before. Make your HypnoBirthing skills work for you, and get rid of the memories of the previous birth or births.

- **Parenting**—Did you learn positive attitudes toward parenting that you feel comfortable with? If not, do you feel less than adequate about your ability to be a good parent? Do you feel overwhelmed? Quite often people who did not grow up with good role models can learn a great deal from less-than-great models about what they wouldn't want to do in their own parenting. Turn it into a positive factor.

- **Support**—Do you feel secure with the support that your partner and/or family will provide? Is there someone who will share the responsibilities of caring for the baby? Sometimes just tackling the issue and letting people know you will want and need support will resolve the matter. In other circumstances, take advantage of the opportunity to see what strengths you must build to effectively provide your own best support.

- **Marriage/relationship**—Is your marriage/relationship secure, loving, and mutually nurturing? Are you confident that your relationship is strong and that it will weather the additional concerns of raising a child? Are there some agreements you need to work out? Have you really "talked"? Perhaps a confidence-building session can help you sort out your abilities. Working together in HypnoBirthing can bring about a stronger bond than you ever believed could exist.

- **Career**—Will you be able to continue to pursue your own goals with reorganising and planning? Will your plans need to be put on hold? Are you ambivalent about going back to work or staying home with your baby? Sorting through these questions can help you reconcile with what you really feel you want to do.

- **Housing**—Is there room in your home, as well as in your heart, for your new baby? Can accommodations be easily made? Can you make changes? If not, express those wishes; and you'll soon see how your circumstances can change.

- **Medical care**—Do you feel comfortable with your present medical care provider? Do you feel that he or she is supportive of your plans for your birthing? Are there lingering doubts? Have you discussed your preferences for a natural birth with this person and made your wishes known? Are your decisions fear-based or confidence-based?

- **Finances**—Do you see finances being "stretched" as a result of adding another person into your life? Ask your HypnoBirthing practitioner about some abundance work. The Law of Attraction can help in this regard: Remember, you get what you say and see.

- **Prior relationships**—Are you carrying around some unhappy memories of an earlier relationship or an experience that has left hurtful thoughts? It's time to eliminate those thoughts and let them go by having a release session.

- **Personal experience of abuse**—Are you harbouring unhappy memories of an experience of physical or sexual abuse? Because these experiences are so associated with your body, bitter or hurtful memories can easily rise to the surface during birthing. Birthing is one of the most profoundly physical experiences you will know in your lifetime. Overwhelming feelings of helplessness, inadequacy, and fear have the ability to make your body shut down or resist. It is important that you do release work with a qualified hypnotherapist before you advance any further into your pregnancy.

Please take this assessment seriously. Your mind and body work best when both are in harmony so that you can approach your birthing as free of limiting thoughts and emotions as possible.

The Power of the Mind

Every thought becomes a plan.
If you think a negative thought or vision, it becomes
a negative prediction; if you think a positive thought or
vision, it becomes a positive prediction and plan.

Marie Mongan

We've just seen the power of the mind, specifically how fear can interrupt the body and the natural birth process. The good news is that the opposite is also true: Positive thought and relaxation can help the body and enhance its ability to birth freely, effectively, and with no ill effects. That is, after all, what HypnoBirthing is all about.

As far back as early Grecian times, relaxation, visualisation, and quiet recitations have been used by priests to aid people in ridding themselves of illnesses. Tribal Indian customs and "old wives" superstitions were used for centuries to bring about physical and emotional healing.

Now, many years later, we are coming to an awareness and acceptance of the ways in which self-hypnosis can physically and chemically affect your body's tissues and mentally reprogramme behaviours that can impede success.

Dr. Bruce Lipton, a well-known author, is in the forefront today with his work on the effect of the mind in changing tissues at the cellular level. Through studies of everything from memory to dreams to subtle eye movements, researchers are discovering that the mind and the images held within it can largely determine your success or failure in life. Motivational consultants, Olympic coaches and other sports trainers, as well as people in medicine, are realising that visualisation—the process of mentally producing pictures of a desired goal or result—is an important factor in the achievement of that goal, and they are routinely incorporating self-hypnosis and visualisation sessions into their programmes.

Educational psychologists have conducted visualisation studies suggesting that extrapolative learning—the method of mentally working through a physical process—can produce a response within muscles that is similar to what would occur if the routine were physically practised.

When in self-hypnosis you visualise your ideal birth scene, it becomes stronger than any of the birth stories and negative comments that you have heard. The brain and nervous system are saturated with a picture of a specific, ideal sensory vision that seems so real it becomes imprinted in the brain. This occurs exactly the way that real experiences become embedded within the memory of the inner-conscious. When a person is in a relaxed state, the mind more easily adapts to the imagery and accepts the suggested vision as being real. The assimilation of the repeated image causes the belief in the desired outcome.

Though neuroscientists are just beginning to understand how this occurs on a cellular level, sufficient study of this phenomenon has resulted in a very clearly defined set of Laws of the Mind. The concept of easier birthing through the positive application of these Laws is changing the view of birthing and is the basis of HypnoBirthing.

The Powerful Laws of the Mind

The application of four specific Laws of the Mind has a direct effect on changing the view of birthing, and these Laws are the basis for much of the work that we do in HypnoBirthing.

The Law of Psycho-Physical Response
The Law of Repetition
The Law of Harmonious Attraction
The Law of Motivation

The Law of Psycho-Physical Response: The Body Follows the Mind

The process of achieving desired results through application of the Laws of the Mind can be more clearly understood by examining the Robot Theory forwarded by Dr. Al Krazner in his book *The Wizard Within*. The Robot Theory is based on the Law of Psycho-Physical Response. This law states that for every suggestion, thought, or emotion one entertains, there is a corresponding physiological and chemical response within the body. This is the most important Law of the Mind in regard to birthing.

According to psychologist Candice Pert, the body is the action component of the mind. What is experienced in the body is determined in the mind. Therefore, what the mind chooses to accept or perceive as being real, the robot body, accordingly, responds to. The mind does not have the ability to act. Therefore, it sends messages to the body demanding action. The body, in turn, plays out the thought. Pavlov's experiment with the dogs that eventually became conditioned to salivate at the ringing of a bell in anticipation of receiving food is perhaps the most commonly recognised example of this mind-body connection.

We experience this law almost every day of our lives. I'm sure it would not be difficult for you to recall any number of incidents when a loud, sudden noise or the unexpected appearance of a person or an object in your path caused you to startle, duck, draw back, or involuntarily cry out.

A dad in one of my classes described experiencing an instant and noticeable physical response when seeing the flashing lights of a police car in his rearview mirror at a time when he was driving well beyond the speed limit. It was not until he pulled over to the side of the road and the policeman continued past him that he became aware of how strong a physiological effect his thoughts had created within his body. He could feel the accelerated pounding of his heart, the dampness accruing at his underarms, the white-knuckle grip he had on the steering wheel, and the long, continuous intake of breath, without exhaling. He was also hugely aware of the relief he felt as he exhaled and his shoulders receded back into the frame of his body. When the mind no longer perceived that he was being threatened, he relaxed back into a state of calm.

Of course, the most obvious example of the psycho-physical response is the one that has brought you to HypnoBirthing class to prepare for your baby's birth—sexual arousal.

When the mind entertains a sexual thought and a subsequent visualisation, the body responds by preparing for the sex act with the male experiencing penile erection and the female experiencing lubrication of the vaginal wall. This all comes naturally, with the robot body acting out the desires of the mind. It is part of the master plan for all reproduction.

Utilising this Law of the Mind so that it works with you and for you, and not against you, during your birthing is essential. If the mind is dwelling on fearful, negative images of birth, the body is thrown unintentionally into a defence mode. The physical response then becomes the antithesis to normal birthing—tension.

You will become skilled in using your own natural abilities to bring your mind and body into psycho-physical harmony so that the thoughts you use in practise are those that will condition your body and your mind to create endorphins—those neuropeptides that create a feeling of well-being. You will learn special deepening techniques that will help you to connect with your baby and work with your body to bring yourself even deeper as your labour advances.

The Law of Repetition

Since repetition is the key to conditioning, the Law of Repetition becomes an important aspect of your preparation. The more you take a single thought and express it mentally or out loud, the more deeply it becomes ingrained in your mind's eye and the more readily the mind accepts it as reality.

Had Pavlov rung the bell once or twice or only on occasion, the dog would not have been able to make the association of the ringing of the bell with receiving food or a treat, and he would not have salivated. Therefore, it is important that you routinely recite the birthing affirmations that your practitioner will provide you in your class and that are recorded on the Rainbow Relaxation CD or MP3 that can be purchased as an accompaniment to this book.

The Law of Harmonious Attraction: The Power of Language

Words and thoughts are powerful and profoundly affect our every-day experiences and beliefs. Equally significant is the harm that is created by the negative energy of the confusing, harsh, and frightening words of conventional birthing.

A second Law of the Mind, the Law of Harmonious Attraction, is very much in evidence here. This law states that what we put out in the way of thinking and speaking creates energy that comes back to us in the same form in subsequent experiences. This is what I call the "echo effect" or the "boomerang effect." Whatever thought or emotion you throw out to the world will come back to you exactly as you first proposed it. Applying this law on a daily basis is important. The best advice, according to Esther Hicks in the Abraham-Hicks Material, is, "If it's not what you're wanting, don't go there."

Words have energy, power, and vibrations that translate into action. Regardless of whether you are the person speaking or the person being spoken to, the sound and vibration of what is being said cause an emotional response within your mind and a physiological and chemi-cal response within your mind-body. Over time, the frequency of that response becomes part of your belief system, strengthening itself each time a similar vibration is accepted. It then attracts more of the same.

Even when we silently engage in self-talk, our words have force. Each time we speak to ourselves in a less-than-complimentary way— "Are you stupid, or what?"—or use similar self-denigrating words, we leave an imprint of inadequacy upon our subconscious.

You can see this demonstrated as you listen to the people around you. Notice that healthy people rarely speak of becoming ill. However, people who are not healthy frequently punctuate their conversation with talk of their physical ailments. Think about the phrase, "The rich get richer, and the poor get poorer." Rich people don't often speak of being poor or not being able to afford goods. On the other hand, poor people, or people who "think poor," regularly end thoughts of spending with the phrase, "I can't afford it." They remain in that situation and go through life affording very little. It is therefore essential that you keep your thoughts and language focused on what you do want rather than creating wasted negative energy around circumstances that you don't want.

The little ditty that you may have heard on the playground when you were a child—"Sticks and stones may break my bones, but names will never hurt me"—may be a good comeback as a temporary defence against words that sting, but, physiologically, it is not true. Caustic, belittling, frightening, and abusive words do, indeed, hurt and can cause a lasting imprint. Tell a baby just learning to walk or beginning to accomplish tasks on his own that he is clumsy or a klutz, and after a while, the child begins to feel clumsy and moves in ways that are clumsy. Tell him that his everyday, normal bodily functions are "smelly and disgusting," and he begins to feel bad about his body and himself for having created a disgusting situation. The negative imprint takes hold, stays with him, and grows. The more potent the thought, the more potent the imprint.

Concepts that you are exposed to repeatedly in many places and from many sources become part of a conditioning that becomes embedded in your thoughts over time. The Law of Repetition governs that process. It is important for you to recognise that frequency does not necessarily equal fact.

The association of pain with childbirth is an example of a universally held conditioning, and it has become the source of needless suffering because of the myths that have grown up around it. By the same token, if you listen to affirmations of positive, gentle birth on a daily basis, it will contribute to positive conditioning.

Words and suggestions set off a chain of feelings, beliefs and reactions that can be uplifting, encouraging, and supportive—or totally debilitating. The following chart shows the flow of energy and the effect of words.

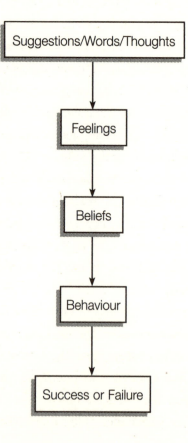

Words create thoughts and emotions; repeatedly entertaining the same thoughts conjures up feelings. Over time, these feelings become beliefs. We begin to act out those beliefs by our behaviour. Our behaviour shapes our experiences. Positive behaviour creates positive experiences; negative behaviour creates negative experiences. Hence, in HypnoBirthing, we focus only on the positive.

For all of these reasons, HypnoBirthing parents learn to use language that more nearly describes what is happening within the birthing mother's body during birth. This gentle language is more meaningful to parents than language that is couched in medical academicism—appropriate for the medical caregivers in communicating with each other, but frightening and potentially harmful to the birthing family.

The language you use and the language you hear from people around you, including caregivers and childbirth educators, keeps your mind in a state of calm, or conversely, triggers a state of unrest, stress, and fear. Learn to choose your words carefully and associate with people who reinforce your own positive thinking about birthing. If you are being bombarded by people who want to tell you birth horror stories, suggest that you wait until after you have your baby to exchange birth stories. Don't get pulled into those kinds of conversations.

This kind of thinking, speaking, and living, as well as the support that you give to each other, will help you to work together toward a positive birth experience. This calmness will be there for you during birthing, and it spills over into every aspect of your family life.

To truly embrace the concept of gentle, normal birth, learn to think and speak in the kinder, softer word substitutes that appear on the list that follows. As you become accustomed to this language, you will become aware of the importance of this mental transition.

HypnoBirthing Language	Medicalised Language
Use:	**Instead of:**
Uterine surge or waves	Contractions
Birth Companion	Coach
Receive the Baby	Catch the Baby
Birth/Birthing	Deliver/Delivery
Birthing Time/Month	Due Date
Pressure/Sensation Tightening	Pain or Contractions
Membranes Release	Water Breaking/Rupturing
Birth Path	Birth Canal
Birth Breathing	Pushing
Special Circumstances	Complications
Uterine Seal	Mucous Plug
Birth Show	Bloody Show
Near Completion/Nearly Complete	Transition
Thinning Opening	Effacing/Dilating
Pre-born/Unborn Baby	Foetus
First-/Second-Time Mum	Primip/Multip
Perineal Rim Unfolds	Perineal Rim Stretches
Parents	Clients/Patients
Pre-Labour Warm-ups	Braxton-Hicks
Pelvic Floor Exercises	Kegels
New Born	Neonate
Resting Labour	Stalled or Shut-down Labour
Practise Labour	False Labour

*Birth-savvy Mothers, who value totally
unmedicated and intervention-free birthing,
have a new term for it—"Pure Birth."*

William and Martha Sears, *The Birth Book*

It is this kind of birth that we refer to as instinctual.

The Law of Motivation: What You Want Is What You Get

The Law of Motivation also affects the physical body's capabilities. We have all read accounts of nearly impossible feats accomplished by people who risked their own lives to save the life of a child. When the mind is highly motivated, the body responds properly.

Consider the football player who sprains an ankle at the beginning of the last quarter of the game. Because his conscious attention and motivation is totally focused on playing the game and winning, he may feel the pressure of the swelling of the ankle but feels no pain. His mind has narrowed its focus and is accepting only the suggestion that he must remain in the game and play his hardest. His ankle does not accept the sharp twist as a source of pain because only the mind is able to think or react to pain stimuli. If there is no pain stimuli, he feels no pain. It is not until the game is over and the motivation to put all of his energy into winning the game is no longer necessary that his mind is directed: the message of the sprain is relayed to the mind, the mind interprets it, and sends it back, and he begins to feel the discomfort.

When we examine motivation to see how it affects the way in which a woman births, we need only to look at a story that received national news coverage several years ago. It involved a very pregnant young woman who was attending a prom when she went into labour. She excused herself, left the dance floor and went into the ladies' room where she proceeded to have her baby, quickly, quietly, and unbeknownst to anyone else. Her fear of being detected created a motivation far stronger than any fear she may have regarding the birth; and she was able to return to the prom activities after only a brief period of labour. Her mind never accepted, or even considered, that there would be any impediments to this birth or that she would experience the long, typical labour that our society has come to expect, especially for a woman having a first baby.

While it is difficult to believe, we sometimes see the reverse of the previous example. If motivation is accompanied by a "secondary benefit," a person can actually bring about what, for most people, would be an unwanted situation—an illness, a bad outcome, a hardship. Without consciously being aware of it, "victims" of the secondary benefit can create circumstances that allow them to accomplish what they consider is a better end, even though it means they endure less than optimal circumstances.

Could the need for attention create motivation for a high-maintenance pregnancy? It definitely can and occasionally does. If a pregnant woman wants and needs to be pampered, "waited upon," and coddled, and buys into the concept that pregnancy is an abnormal condition and she is "ill," the attention that she gains during a troublesome pregnancy and a difficult birthing can definitely make it all worthwhile in her mind. She barely tolerates her pregnancy and constantly proclaims her annoyance at all the aches, pains, and other pregnancy "disorders," while she uses body language that demonstrates her plight. Family members often contribute to this scenario by cautioning the woman that she must "give in" to her frailty during this precarious time of her life.

Several years ago, a mum came to my classes talking about the horrendously long and difficult births her mother and all of the women in her family experienced. This was the centrepiece of her conversation week after week. As I got to know her family, I saw that all the women in the family talked in "victim" language. In spite of the fact that their birth stories were horrific, they were delighted to tell all of the details, each one surpassing the other, and each rushing in to grab her opportunity to tell how bad her pregnancies and birthings were. The mum and dad appeared to embrace the HypnoBirthing philosophy, but I was not surprised that her birthing story was one that could easily match and top those of her family members. The drama surrounding the birth was incredible, and there was a gathering of family and friends invited in to observe the performance. It was more important for this young woman to be able to remain in good standing in the sorority of her family and friends than it was to remain outside the group and to birth her baby calmly and peacefully as she had prepared.

This is not to say that all labours that are drawn out and difficult have behind them some secondary benefit. Nevertheless, it is important to assess your own motivation and intent as you approach your birthing and consider, in light of all we've spoken of here, how you will apply these Laws of the Mind so that they work for you.

Motivation is closely tied to your intent and your self-image. It is said that a woman births pretty much the same way that she lives life. For that reason, it is imperative that you take the time to do an assessment of how you see yourself and whether this image is productive for you or counterproductive. Much of the determining aspects of how you will make important choices concerning your birthing are factored on how you regard birth and your own role in this experience.

Two models—the whole-person model and the dependent model—determine how you will approach your pregnancy and birthing. Review each model and evaluate which traits you want to strengthen and expand upon as you make important decisions regarding your baby and your birthing. The model you choose to follow will be invaluable to you as you continue your adventure into pregnancy, birthing, and lifelong parenting.

Dependent Model	Whole-Person Model
uninformed/unknowing	knowledgeable
submissive	powerful
passive onlooker	involved
conforming	forward thinking
reconciled	fulfilled
easily led	directing
vulnerable	trusting
helpless	self-sufficient
vacillating	decisive
threatened	confident
embarrassed	assertive
resigned	satisfied

Understanding Self-Hypnosis

There is a considerable amount of misinformation and a terrible lack of good information surrounding self-hypnosis. This is because the only exposure that many people have had to hypnosis, in general, is what they've seen as entertainment—stage hypnosis. Without going into detail, I will simply remind you that the people who are on the stage during a stage show are volunteers, there to have a good time. Since all hypnosis is self-hypnosis, it is easy for them to accept the roles that the hypnotist suggests to them. They're having fun.

Contrary to what is portrayed in movies and literature, it is impossible to cause someone to do something that is against his morals or his principles while he is participating in hypnosis. If a suggestion were to be made that is contrary to any value that a person holds, the person would immediately revert to an alert state and refuse to carry out the directive.

What many people may not know is that hypnosis is being used to benefit people in many medical, dental, and therapeutic applications. Hypnosis is widely used to help people release fears, overcome the discomfort of the effects of chemotherapy, prepare for surgery, stop stuttering, end nail-biting, and a host of other annoying habits. Hypnosis is so effective that it was recognised in 1957 by the American Medical Association as a beneficial therapy for many physical and emotional needs.

Hypnosis is a very natural state that most of us exist in during a large part of our day. When we become engrossed with our work and lose track of time or of what is going on around us, that is hypnosis. We are in a hypnotic state when we get caught up in daydreams or become so immersed in a movie or a television show that we emotionally react to what the actors are experiencing.

When you are in hypnosis during your labour, you'll be able to hear conversations and may or may not wish to join in. Though you will be totally relaxed, you will also be fully in control. To the person who is not familiar with self-hypnosis, you may even appear as though you've taken some kind of medication to put you into this profoundly relaxed state. During your birthing you will be aware of your uterine surges, but you will experience them comfortably and with the knowledge that you are very much in charge. You'll be able to interrupt your relaxation whenever you wish and resume it whenever you wish.

As your labour moves nearer to birth, you will most likely choose to go even deeper within to your birthing body and your baby so that together you can work in harmony through birth. Though you will not be able to visually experience it, you will be able to physically know that your baby is very much a birth partner in this adventure. When you are tuned into your body, you will sense and know exactly what you and your baby are doing.

You'll become skilled in using your own natural abilities to bring your mind and body into perfect harmony. You will gain an understanding of the physiology of labour that goes beyond what is usually taught in other classes. You will learn special relaxation conditioning and labour techniques that will enable you to connect with and work with your body and your baby as you experience labour. The repetitive practise of these techniques will make it possible for you to instantly achieve this relaxation and maintain it for as long as you wish through labour.

The value of self-hypnosis comes from learning to reach that level of mind where suggestions that you give yourself effectively influence your physiological experience. Your HypnoBirthing practitioner will help you learn to reach this level, where you focus only on calm and comfort. You will see, hear, and practise these techniques in class and will be given practise tapes or CDs that you will work with on a daily basis at home. Your birth companion will also be given scripts to use when you practise together two or three times a week.

There is no magic benefit that accrues from just coming to classes. You must be willing to apply the practice that is required to reach these levels of relaxation that will be there for you when you are in labour.

These skills will be applicable to many facets of your life, as well as for the birthing of your child. Many couples find that the months of preparation in relaxation benefit them in the way they deal with day-to-day situations and have a positive effect on how they interact with each other. A mother who was in one of my classes said, "I came to HypnoBirthing to learn how to have a baby, and I learned how to have a life." It's that powerful if you learn to utilise it.

Relaxation also has a calming effect upon the baby. "Mellow" is the word many parents use when describing their babies. We like to think they are "better natured."

Falling in Love with Your Baby

*Leave it to a baby to turn your world
upside down, take your breath away and make you
fall in love again. With his toothless grin,
your baby sets your heart on fire.*

Jan Blaustone, *The Joy of Parenthood*

We know that calm, soothing thoughts and emotions have a bearing on the way in which you bring your baby into the world. Love is one of the most important emotions in helping to build a positive anticipation—the love that you as parents feel for each other and the love that you actively share with the baby that you are carrying.

When is the best time for you to fall in love with your baby? If you haven't already fallen madly in love with your baby and are not playing and communicating with her on a daily basis, now is the time. Getting acquainted with your baby is a very magical experience, and you don't have to wait until she is born to enjoy making this connection.

Once your baby is born, you wouldn't think of going about your daily routine without making time for frequent breaks that are especially devoted to talking, playing, and loving her. Babies have a way of drawing that kind of attention from family members and strangers alike. No one can resist their magnetic charm—so compelling it can bring activities and conversation to a screeching halt.

You can begin to connect socially and emotionally with your unborn baby as soon as you know that you are pregnant. In addition to making your pregnancy so much more enjoyable and exciting, when you "tune in" to this little person who has become part of your life, you lay the foundation for a relationship that can last for the rest of your lives. Pre-birth parenting activities tell your baby that he is welcome and wanted.

The idea that both parents influence their pre-born baby is neither supposition nor superstition. The close bond that is built while the baby is still in the womb can be very real when it is time to connect with your baby during birthing.

Thanks to the relatively young study of foetology, advanced during the late seventies and early eighties by Dr. Thomas Verny in his book *The Secret Life of the Unborn Child,* we know that babies are cognizant during their time in the womb. All of baby's womb life is actually his first classroom. There he learns lessons and develops emotionally, physically, spiritually, and socially. Parents should do all they can to be sure that the baby's emotional development, his sense of well-being, and his esteem as a loved being are being fostered through caring and consistent pre-birth parenting.

The nine months that the baby spends in the womb are nine months of growth and development for parents as well. They learn the importance of evolving as a family, and mums learn the importance of planning and working, together with their babies, toward achieving the goal of a gentle birth for both baby and mother.

Dr. David Chamberlain, author of *Babies Remember Birth,* later published as *The Mind of Your Newborn Baby,* spent many years investigating the effects of birth trauma upon a baby. He states that babies are active participants in birth, and they do remember their birth experience. The imprint of that experience is carried throughout their lives. All one has to do is gaze into the alert, knowing eyes of a newborn who has not been drugged during her journey into being, and it is immediately evident that there is a lot of thought going on. Without saying a word, the baby transmits a message: "I know."

Pre- and perinatal psychology is a branch of research that focuses on the effects of environment upon the baby as he is developing within the womb and during the birthing experience. Ongoing study is attempting to determine the degree to which a baby in the uterus is affected by the environment in which he is living and the manner in which his parents interact with him and each other.

While we know that everything the mother puts into her body crosses the placenta and affects the baby, this is also true of emotions. When we offer the pre-born baby love, play, and music, we reinforce his positive feelings of security. On the negative side, it's been found that the pulse rate of the unborn baby rises abruptly when the baby is exposed to screaming, yelling, loud or disturbing noises, and emotional upsets. Be aware of the kind of environment and experiences you are providing for your unborn baby.

It is so important that dads get involved in nurturing both mother and baby and that mothers recognise the need for nurturing both dad and baby. Reciprocal nurturing of one parent for the other sends a strong message of security to their pre-born baby: This is a loving family.

As a result of Verny's studies, and those of his colleagues, it was found that babies in the womb react to stimuli outside of the uterus. Intentionally initiating certain kinds of interaction and love-play can result in positive prenatal, perinatal, and postnatal bonding.

Findings suggest that babies within the womb react to vibrations, stroking, tapping, rubbing, squeezing, conversation, voices, music, light, heat, cold, pressing to simulate the birth experience, teasing, loud noises, TV sounds, and humor.

Babies who were exposed to soft music and singing during their time in the womb were calmer, happier, and better adjusted to life outside of the womb. It is also believed that they are better sleepers. Babies love the sound of their parents' voices, especially when they are sung to. Some mothers report that while singing to their pre-born babies, the babies responded with a gentle moving action. Music has vibration that babies are sensitive to. If the vibration is gentle and calming, they have a feeling of well-being.

Dr. Michael Lazarev, a leading Russian paediatrician, emphasises the importance of helping the baby to become familiar with musical sounds. He concluded that if you listen to your unborn baby, he will let you know what activities and sounds he prefers.

In a study at the University of Salzburg, mothers who developed a real sense of being connected with their pre-born babies and who interacted with the babies in talk and play tended to view their bodies with an air of pride and fully accepted their increasing size as a natural part of the development of the baby. Fathers who were involved in bonding displayed the same kind of awe with respect to the shape of the mother's body and the development taking place inside. There was a respect for the life being carried in the womb. Overall, their pregnancies seemed to be easier, as were their birthings. They approached birthing with a relaxed confidence. Later, both parents seemed to adopt a softer, more balanced attitude toward caregiving. Parents displayed greater feelings of enjoyment, love, and respect for each other and for the baby.

The benefits to babies were also profound. There were fewer premature births and fewer low-birthweight babies. Reports showed a noticeable increase in the socialisation of the babies who experienced pre-birth parenting. Overall health and weight gain were very positive. HypnoBirthing parents tell us that their young babies hardly cry and are exceptionally alert.

I believe that one of the most important advantages of pre-birth parenting to the baby is that when parents truly connect in attitude as a family prior to the birth of the baby, they accept the responsibility for planning and directing their births. They are as committed to ensuring the safety and comfort of the baby during its journey into the world as they are when their baby is part of their family outside the womb. I also believe that pre-birth parenting helps them become practised in accepting the responsibility of parenting later.

Knowing that the baby is fully aware of its surroundings and the people who are his parents, it is only reasonable that the baby also thrives when there is interaction and socialisation with the people with whom he lives.

Recommendations for Pre-Birth Parenting

- Learn the suggested relaxation techniques and practise them daily—baby needs peace too. Since baby is aware, he is listening to the music and calming suggestions at the same time as his mum.

- Play with baby physically—sway, sway, sway; dance, dance, dance; rub, rub, rub; pat, pat, pat; squeeze, squeeze, squeeze; press, press, press (all done gently).

- Use guided imagery and visualisation. (See the Birth Companion's Reading and Rainbow Relaxation in this book, as well as the Pre-Birth Parenting CD.)

- Carry on conversations with baby—say affirmations, read stories with animation and imitation of animal sounds, play children's tapes.

- While relaxing in the tub, massage your belly with lukewarm water and sing or talk to your baby.

- Play soothing music—sounds of ocean, birds, wind, soft piano, guitar, madrigals, flute, harp, nature sounds, and animal sounds—so that baby develops a wider awareness of these things.

- Have family and friends greet and interact with baby.

- Put yourself in the baby's frame of reference—how wholesome are the surrounding noises, voices, attitudes, emotions, foods, temperatures, air, odours?

Prenatal Bonding Exercises

Important facets of the HypnoBirthing programme are the discussions and exercises for parents that help them to truly connect and fall in love with their pre-born baby. These activities help the parents develop a sensitivity to how the baby perceives his surroundings and often cause them to evaluate how their lifestyle, their emotional well-being, and their relationship with each other can impact the baby's emotional development and sense of feeling loved and secure.

The exercises on the HypnoBirthing Pre-Birth Parenting CD are valuable relaxation lessons and image-building tools for both parents. These activities help them develop a stronger sense of their own self-worth, as well as serve as meditations that will help them bond with their pre-born baby. The time spent with these guided images may prove to be among the most valuable gifts that you can give to yourself and your baby.

Another way to establish a connection with your baby and to explore his world is to take part in the following exercise. We call it "Be the Baby" because we ask you to imagine yourself in the role of the baby in the womb, experiencing what life is like for the baby.

As the practitioner leads you through this exercise, take advantage of the opportunity to think about how your unborn baby might respond to these questions and how you can begin to actively do things that will enhance the baby's feeling of being loved and wanted.

Be the Baby Exercise

What your baby perceives—what she accepts and embraces while in the uterus—becomes part of her essence and identity and forms the creation of a conscious ego that accepts, caresses, and acknowledges its own true self.

Imagine that you are the baby developing within your mother's womb, listening to conversations, experiencing your surroundings, absorbing emotions and moods of those around you. Reflect for a few minutes on how you feel as that child who will soon be born into your family.

- To what degree are your parents spending time in relaxation practise to help ensure a calm birth for you?

- How welcome do you feel? Do you already feel that you are part of the family?

- How loved do you feel? Do people talk to you with love each day?

- What kinds of messages are you receiving from things that are said about you?

- How do you feel about the way your parents interact with each other?

- What kind of pace do your parents keep? Do you feel sure there will be time purposely created for you as you're growing up?

- What kind of atmosphere will you come into? Peaceful? Loving? Caring? Happy?

- How confident are you that you will be raised with love and patience?

- How calm a world is being prepared for you?

- How kind and loving are the people you will be living with?

- Do you feel that your parents will do what is necessary to ensure your gentle entry into the world?

- Do your parents talk in gentle, loving ways?

- Is each motion that you make received with joy?

- What kinds of sounds/music/noises do you live with?

- Are you being provided with the best nourishing food to help you grow and develop in a strong, healthy way?

- How wholesome is the air that you are breathing? Will it foster good health for you?

- Is your environment and your body free of smoke, alcohol, and drugs?

- How certain are you that you will be helped and guided toward becoming a loved and loving human being?

- What kind of assurance do you have that your parents will give you understanding as you learn to adjust to your strange, new world?

- Are you confident that you will learn by guidance, not punishment?

Take a moment now to quietly connect with your baby. Ask your baby to tell you what it is that she might like to add to this list. Is there a message that your baby has for you? What would make her feel more loved, more secure?

Reflecting on your responses to these questions, are there some changes that you feel you can make in your baby's environment? Are there some resolutions that you, as parents, need to think about and adopt?

We recommend these activities for creating lasting expressions of welcome for your baby:

- Write letters to the baby or keep a journal expressing your delight that he will soon be here. Save letters to present to the child later.

- Take pregnancy photographs of mother, as well as mother and dad together.

- Record messages to your baby on a tape or CD in addition to letters.

- Videotape your birthing, complete with a birthing-day message given to the baby during labour.

- Videotape siblings talking and listening to the baby or telling the baby a story.

- Involve siblings in decorating baby's room and take pictures.

- Start a scrapbook and includes pictures that show how your body is changing as the baby develops, as well as special events like a visit from grandparents, trips to memorable places, a baby shower, a mother-baby luncheon, or a blessing way.

The Power and Art of
Doing Nothing

This chapter on experiencing a beautiful, calm, and tranquil birth while doing absolutely nothing will pull together all of the facets of this programme that you have already studied with those parts of the programme, particularly the birth, which is yet to come. It includes the rationale behind the previous chapters—the educational component, philosophy, the breathing techniques, the history of how we got to where we are, the ways of preparing your body and your mind and relaxation with the parts of the programme that are yet to come, i.e., the actual birthing experience.

To understand the connection between birthing and "doing nothing" we must first address a topic that is more commonly related to animals in nature.

What we are talking about here is something that is not often attributed to human mothers, but is more commonly related when we speak of animal mothers in nature. What we are suggesting is that you look within the gifts that nature has already bestowed upon you—collectively called instinct.

Are You Out of Your Mind?

It is futile for you to attempt to direct your body. While we do spend time teaching you breathing styles that will assist you to relax to the point where you can quiet your mind, we do not attempt to teach you how to use your mind to keep your birthing on target. Just the opposite is true. We teach you how to keep your mind out of the way while you do nothing but allow yourself to completely relax. With the help of your natural instinct, the perfect physiological order and design of your reproductive system will carry you through your entire birthing. If your keep your mind clear of chatter filled with questions, doubts, instructions, and techniques intended to teach your body how to birth, it will happen on its own. Without this interference of your mind-talk, your natural instincts will take over for you. Not anything or anyone knows better than your own instinct.

Of course, we know that there are devices, apparatuses, and drugs that forcefully make your body do what it already knows how to do. But how dare we presume to attempt to improve upon what nature has perfectly orchestrated and validated over centuries?

Dr. Michel Odent, world-renowned birth professional states, "You cannot improve upon a natural function. The answer is not to hinder it."

In presenting your relaxation session, we suggest you give your body permission to take the lead, not the other way around.

If we examine the definition of instinct, we find that the words and phrasing related to instinct all suggest activity that occurs naturally without thought or initiation.

Here are some words and phrases related to instinct:

spontaneous impulse	action not self-initiated
inner sense	reflex
compulsion	predisposition

A knowing that it is not based on experience or learning

A natural, inherent tendency to make a complex and specific
response to stimuli without involving reason

All these words indicate that the body is capable of functioning and reacting to situations without your conscious thought or consent or input. Some everyday situations that call for involuntary action would be:

- When you attempt to maintain balance.

- When you cower or use your hands to protect yourself from an object hurtling toward you.

- When you pull back your hand from an object that is burning hot.

- When you startle at a sudden loud noise.

When instinct is used to complete a natural body function, these occurrences are naturally set in place while "nothing" is needed to initiate them. Why then are birthing women asked to believe and accept that somehow the beasts in the animal kingdom are endowed with this gift of instinct, while human mothers are somehow overlooked?

You may not have given it a great deal of thought along the way, but you've been depending upon nature and instinct throughout your life, even before you were born. When you were in the womb, no one taught you that when your bladder was full, you needed to do something to release the urine that you were accumulating. Your bladder just released the urine into the amniotic sac. You did nothing to make it happen.

From the moment that you emerged, you took your first breath. Who taught you how to take that breath? You did absolutely nothing to make it happen. Had you been allowed and assisted, you would have instinctively made your way to your mother's breast to feed, as do all mammals. It is no accident that the scent of colostrum is the same as that of amniotic fluid.

Over time as you grew and developed, with nothing to tell you how or when, you used your own special form of communication to let your parents know that you were hungry or needed a little extra comforting. When you felt secure, you could fall asleep in your parent's loving arms. What did you do to learn to fall asleep or to awaken? That's right—nothing.

Fast-forward to when you were a teenager. Your body changed with nothing but internal hormonal secretions to act as catalysts—you became a woman. The Power of Nothing was, and has been, alive in your human experiences in so many ways, and it is ready to perform this magnificent task easily and adeptly. You found yourself in tune with your body and knew its signals.

Nothing had to teach you that you were experiencing your first love. You instinctively knew it and felt it. And when the time was right, you needed nothing to teach you how to express that love physically.

But here we are today, you are pregnant or planning to become pregnant, and all of a sudden it seems that you require advice and counseling from all directions. You are bombarded by well-intentioned friends and family who feel the need to tell their birth stories.

You learn from your care providers and all the experts and women who have birthed a baby that your body is flawed.

You learn that you must place your trust and power into the hands of others. Your previous trust and confidence in yourself as a vital healthy woman quickly crumbles. All of society views you as fragile, vulnerable, and hopelessly emotional.

Abraham Maslow (an American psychologist best known for his theory of a hierarchy of innate human needs) would argue that all these occurrences that pregnant women experience are necessary because human mothers have lost their ability to call upon their birthing instincts. How then do we explain the well-documented fact that since 2009 in the United States alone, seven women in complete comas have given birth to babies unassisted? Their instinct was alive and well and allowed them to birth, in some cases, without being noticed.

HypnoBirthing takes exception to the notion that human mothers have lost their power of instinct. Actually, human mothers have not lost their instinct but have in fact been taught how to birth within the standard medical system.

You will further learn that many of the protocols and procedures that now surround birth are totally contrary to natural, normal means of birthing. One has only to witness that period within a birth when it is time for the baby's descent down through the birth path to total emergence to see that there is little or no allowance for instinct.

It is at this point when care providers are telling mothers that they can now assist and help themselves to birth their babies when just the opposite is true. Complete opening and thinning of the cervix ushers in an entirely new approach. Additional staff are now introduced to the birthing room, the bed on which the mother has been calmly labouring in deep relaxation is "broken down," and mother is directed to "scooch her bottom" to the very end of the bed. Her legs are lifted onto grooved metal stirrups or her knees are held by her birth partner or an attendant up and back toward her shoulders. It's common for hospital staff to become genuinely enthusiastic when you near completion of this phase, as they anticipate your actively "pushing" your baby down to crowning.

From this position the mother is expected by most people in the room to begin to forcefully push her baby into the world, using what is known as the Valsalva manoeuvre, all the while with staff almost rhythmically coaching her with loud voices to, "Keep it comin, keep it comin, keep it comin," or "Push harrrrd!!!" This can continue for as long as two-plus hours while both mother and baby become exhausted. At some point the woman is asked to stop pushing because the baby's head has emerged and baby gets his first impression of his new world.

With a few more surges, baby's body usually emerges on its own. Frequently, however, the baby is pulled from his mother's vaginal outlet. Hardly a scene that reflects instincts associated with birthing.

Aside from all the lessons she is learning about how to birth her baby as directed, the birthing mother soon realises that in spite of all her preparation, she has lost the calm and gentle birth she envisioned. She also becomes aware that she has been stripped of her dignity.

Sadly, doctors, too, have been taught to birth in ways that totally exclude instinct. Many graduates go into practise never having seen a normal, instinctive, and unmedicated birth.

Even more regrettable is that some medical schools are advocating that birth can best be accomplished by removing the baby surgically from its mother. Not too many years ago, the local evening news in a metropolitan city featured interviews with medical students who were to graduate within a few days. One woman announced her specialty: obstetrics. When asked why she chose obstetrics, she replied, "Because

I always wanted to be a surgeon." One can only wonder how her statistics read today.

Why We Don't Push— There's a Kinder Way

"Pushing your baby out" is a rude concept that has no place in gentle birthing; though there are occasions when it becomes necessary to move the birth along more quickly. Pushing is usually counterproductive and is actually a detriment, causing the vaginal sphincters to close ahead of the descending baby. It creates an atmosphere of stress for all involved. Very recent studies suggest that forced pushing over a long period of time can be harmful to a birthing mother and do damage to her pelvic floor. Because the mother is asked to hold her breath and push, the baby is then deprived of much-needed oxygen causing a change in baby's heart rate.

Completion of the opening phase doesn't need to mean the onslaught of a sudden flurry of activity, confusion, or additional staff on the scene. It is important that you avoid any attempt to force or rush this stage. The descent of your baby can be experienced as calmly as your first stage of labour. Many times, HypnoBirthing mums just allow this phase to begin almost unnoticed, as they remain in the position of their choice and just allow the birthing phase to play out, calmly and gently. Because there is no noticeable change in your behaviour, only the most trained eye will detect that you are birthing your baby.

The moves that fall into place at this time should follow the requests you expressed in your birth preferences. You don't want to find yourself caught up in procedures that are different from what you have anticipated or those that your natural instinct dictates.

The material in the chapter—The Law of Natural Birthing Physiology —will clearly show how relying only on nature's gifts, in total relaxation, will allow you to experience the calm and gentle birth of your vision by doing nothing more than what you normally do as you practise your breathing and deepening exercises.

So when it is suggested that you are out of your mind to attempt to birth naturally, you can confidently smile and reply, "Yes, isn't wonderful?"

The Law of
Natural Birthing Physiology

Y ou've explored the Laws of the Mind, as well as the psycho-
physical laws, and you've read how important it is to "empty
your cup," so to speak, to release any and all fears and limiting
thoughts. You've learned that negative thoughts can stand as obstacles
to the confidence you've been building in your ability to birth your
baby as nature intended. Only when your cup is empty can you make
room for new positive thoughts and the real truth about giving birth
instinctively. This chapter will discuss the gifts that nature has already
provided to you to ensure a natural birth. It will tell you what happens
without any effort on your part, but more important, you will learn the
details of *how* and *why* birth can be accomplished instinctively. It will
assure you that there is a precise design, and you are not on your own.

While relaxation, release, and positive affirmations are essential
to your birth preparation, becoming familiar with nature's gifts and
educating yourself to the ways in which your own body and your
baby are fully capable of performing this magnificent task is equally
important. Those nagging fears can be dismissed when you know that

the precise design of nature has already taken care of those issues for you in many surprising ways.

The physical natural functions behind what is happening in labour are not generally discussed. Most women know only that "What happens next" includes the information that their babies will descend down the birth path, crown, and then emerge past the perineum. But they don't know what is in place to help that descent go smoothly and comfortably. They inhibit the journey by using activities that they've been mistakenly taught. The details of what is happening are glossed over. Some of these gifts for birth have occurred already along the way of your pregnancy as your baby was growing and developing. Others are specific to your labour and birth.

There is nothing that you have to do to activate the inner body workings of instinctive birthing. Nature has freely provided you and your baby with these incredible birthing gifts. Relax and learn how and why your birthing plays out smoothly and easily.

The Body Begins to Prepare for Birth at Conception—

Nature has provided for the calm and gentle birth of your baby in many ways that most pregnant women are not made aware of. These gifts are naturally well designed, in physiological ways in which your body and your baby work together to help make birthing easier. Several of these manifestations are subtle and start almost from the very beginning of your pregnancy. Some of them will continue after birth. Others occur at various times during pregnancy and labour, and still others come into play only during labour.

The most welcome of the gifts are those that come during the birthing phase of labour. Because of media portrayal of birth and the profusion of unpleasant birth stories, this phase is the one that birthing mothers seem to fear most. Becoming acquainted with these physiological gifts of nature will allay your fears and boost your confidence.

Formation of the Uterine Seal

After the mother's egg is fertilised and the egg cells begin to divide and develop, the egg makes its way through the fallopian tube down into the upper portion of the uterus. The egg sends out little pseudo pods, which attach the egg to the side of the endometrium. Now, here is the remarkable part. At the instant that the egg has successfully attached to the wall of the uterus, the uterine seal begins to form down at the cervix. At this point the cervix is long, thick, and closed and, along with the uterine seal, will remain that way until just before the start of labour. This seal protects the developing baby from exposure to any bacteria that could otherwise enter the uterus. The uterine seal remains intact until it releases at the beginning of labour.

Early Effects from Hormonal Changes

Almost from the beginning of pregnancy, hormones are secreted that change your cervix from a hard, cartilaginous substance into a substance that is loose, spongy, and pliable. The opening of the cervix is one of the processes of labour that women dread because they think it is a serious cause of pain. You can allay that fear and learn just how effective the hormonal change is by feeling the same cartilaginous stiffness at the end of your nose and then feeling the soft supple substance at the end of your earlobe. Over time, the same transformation happens to allow your cervix to open easily. When you are relaxed during the first phase of your labour and endorphins are flowing, your thinning and opening phase moves along more quickly.

Relaxation

Pregnant or not, your body takes its prompts from your mind. Through your pregnancy, you learn to prepare for your birthing by releasing, relaxing, and letting go. There is not much to learn. If all is going nicely, you actually are doing nothing. You will see from the other gifts that trusting the perfectly designed plan of nature will help you to release and relax. You cannot force relaxation, and only you can bring it on. The relaxation that you experience on a daily basis teaches you to become conditioned to instantly relax your body and to enjoy the euphoric comfort that endorphins provide. Relaxation is one of the most important ways to prepare for birth. This is especially true if you are using a programme with a birth companion or friend or reciting a script especially designed to educate you further about your birthing. Relaxation works because of the way in which your mind works. The mind doesn't know the difference between reality and fantasy. Like a child, your mind accepts a message it receives repeatedly; and, over time, it comes to accept that message as being true. It then works toward the goal. Here we see that Law of Repetition in play.

Endorphin Release

Relaxation is the safest and most effective comfort measure that you will use during birthing. The rapid release of endorphins is particularly prevalent if you have practised deep relaxation and deepening techniques on a daily basis.

Since the constrictor hormone—catecholamine—cannot co-exist with the "feel good hormones"—endorphins—the goal is to reach a state of relaxation from the very start of labour to preclude the secretion of catecholamine. After a while, this focused awareness of being able to reach these deeper levels brings on a feeling of being steeped in the almost buoyant state that is created when larger amounts of endorphins are secreted. Endorphins multiply themselves, so the more you reach deeper levels of relaxation, the more your body will seek that level of relaxation, and you are able to attain it in a shorter amount of time. This natural state of euphoria will gradually become addictive, and you'll find yourself looking forward to each session.

Baby, too, experiences the benefits of daily calm and peace, and his temperament is affected in a positive way. When endorphins are present during labour, the secretion of catecholamine is inhibited; and your body releases the exact amount of oxytocin to cause the birthing muscles to function as they should. With this perfect formula in place, you are able to birth without discomfort, and so is your baby. Because there is no obstructing tension, your birth is able to move along easily and naturally and within a shorter time frame.

As you advance in your pregnancy, you are able to cultivate a deeper trust in instinctive birthing because you are accessing the knowledge of the already-functioning mechanism that is in place within your body. It is a lack of understanding and/or fear that causes constricted birthing muscles. With an ample supply of both knowledge and understanding, you can allow your mind to step aside as you follow, rather than try to lead, the rhythm and flow of your labour that makes all of this possible.

Parents regularly tell us that their babies are mellow and calm and easy to care for during those first few months when they are making the adjustment to life outside the womb. The vertex turn is an early indication of the benefits of remaining stress free through your pregnancy.

Vertex Turn

Between the thirty-second and thirty-seventh week of your pregnancy, your baby will most likely turn into the vertex position, with his head down in preparation for birthing. Because the brain is housed within the baby's skull, the head is the heaviest part of the body. And, therefore, it usually responds readily to the pull of gravity.

Engagement

As soon as the baby's body turns down, engagement can occur. The studies have shown that when you remain upbeat, rather than uptight, throughout your pregnancy and you teach yourself to avoid stress, your baby is also relaxed and upbeat. She is also developing a calm manner and is better able to respond to events and situations that will carry over into her life outside of the womb. Sometimes babies will not turn until well into that thirty-seventh week. There is no cause for alarm if this is the case. Don't allow yourself to be unnecessarily anxious, and don't start anticipating alternative birthing procedures. The vertex turn is an early indication of the benefits of remaining stress free through your pregnancy.

Two or three weeks before the baby is due to be born, he may move down to a point where the widest part of his head will be at the widest part of the midsection of the pelvis. When this occurs, the baby's head is said to be engaged. This is a good sign, though your walking pattern may change, and sitting may become a whole different experience.

Relaxin Release

The hormone relaxin is secreted during the latter part of pregnancy and contributes to normal birthing in a number of ways. It allows the walls of your vagina to become lubricated, to expand, and to become smooth. It assists in softening the lower segment of your uterus and the expansion of the pelvic region.

1. It causes ligaments within your baby's body to relax, and the baby's body becomes more flexible and supple for easier descent and emergence.

2. It weakens the amniotic membrane and allows it to release.

3. It loosens the mother's skeletal ligaments, allowing the front pubic bone (the pubis symphasis) to shift forward to facilitate an easier descent through the birth path to crowning. (This can also cause a change in your walking pattern that makes wearing sensible shoes a must to help avoid falls or sprains.)

Prostaglandins

When you are nearing your birthing time, you may experience a small amount of pre-labour opening. Many women do. In order for this to happen, your body secretes prostaglandins, which eventually trigger oxytocin, which initiates the start of labour. Oxytocin, in turn, causes uterine surges to begin, and it releases the uterine seal. The appearance of the birth show from the release of the seal is one more signal that the onset of labour is near.

Uterine Surge or Wave

Uterine surges or uterine waves are another result of the effects of the presence of oxytocin. During a surge, the longitudinal, or vertical muscles, in perfect precision, smoothly draw the lower horizontal muscles up and out of the way of the baby's head like an ocean wave. It draws back and then gently nudges the baby forward slightly until the cervix is short, thin, and open. The surges then propel the baby out of the cervix and into the birth path. As this happens, another gift of nature often sets in. Surges rest for a while, and mother and baby also rest. There is nothing to be alarmed about if your labour rests. Your labour has not "shut down." Your body is simply resting. If all is well with your baby, do not be pressured into beginning to "push to get things going." If you're not having surges, you should not be prompted to push. Rest and be thankful for the break. Your labour will start again when baby is ready.

Time Distortion

By being relaxed and focused you may lose track of time—this is another welcome feature for both the opening and thinning phase, as well as the birthing phase when baby is descending.

You may decide to doze during this period, which will help the effect of time distortion. Even if you are not asleep, you will look as though you are. This is where you call upon the deeper relaxation levels and use the Power of Nothing, where you go into your birthing body and let your body birth your baby. You may be aware of the downward motion of the baby, and you will experience a full, bulging feeling at the perineum when the baby is crowning. While the descent may seem to take a long time to onlookers, you will hardly be aware of the passing of time. In many cases the reason for that is that with instinctive birthing, nature often does her job more quickly.

Nature's Birth Journey

The journey that your baby takes down through the birth path to crowning and ultimately to emergence is one of the most feared and actually dreaded phases of birthing. This is unfortunate and needless. I say "needless" because fear of this phase is unwarranted. There is no pathological reason for pain in this second phase of birthing. The media has cast a shadow over the joy, excitement, and anticipation that a mother feels during her pregnancy, and it can affect her level of confidence during birthing.

Harbouring fear of this phase is truly unnecessary because it is precisely at the actual birthing time that nature steps in and takes over the course of your labour. You should remain doing nothing. Nature is in charge and assumes management, unless you are thwarted by other means of management from external sources. Of all of the gifts of birthing, the ones provided during the birthing itself are the most remarkable.

Nature's Gifts for the Birth Phase

The Amnesiac State

Toward the end of the thinning and opening phase of your birthing, just before you reach completion, you will sense a feeling of even deeper relaxation drift over you. Through this period you may even feel a deeper connection with your baby. You will forego conversation and just melt into your birthing body. Many women speak of being better able to connect with their babies' downward movement, and they experience a stronger connection with what is happening within them. In those brief moments as the baby nears birth, you may hear people around you, but you definitely will not care to engage in conversation or take part in any activity other than birthing with your baby. We would like to claim that this ultimate relaxation stems from something that you've learned in your HypnoBirthing classes, but this is purely nature's instinctive birthing. All we've done to assist you in this is to teach you how to easily slip into this ultimate state and provide you with the brief script to learn how to do it. So simple.

As your labour advances, you redirect your mind to your birthing body and go within to birth with your baby. It is a very comfortable state where you find you are so relaxed that you don't really care to speak. It will seem as though it takes too much effort to remain in contact with others. You will be able to hear what is happening and you can choose to listen in, or you can shut out noises or conversation entirely, or you can even drift in and out of this state. You can be selective in tuning out all but your birth companion's voice, as the companion prompts you to begin to relax even deeper.

Dr. Gregory White explodes the myth of chaos and pain in this period of descent. Dr. White says:

1. *"The Second Stage is easier: When the mouth of the womb is completely open, the baby begins to slide into the birth canal. The mother begins to feel heavy pressure on the rectum, as though she were about to have a large bowel movement. This is the phase in which there is no physiological reason for discomfort.*

2. *The mother appears to be markedly indifferent to and withdrawn from what is going on around her, although she is not unconscious; she hears everything that is said. Usually, the mother is calmer and more purposeful during the second stage."* (This is the amnesiac state that we in HypnoBirthing *refer to.)*

Fontanels

There have been many jokes and frightening comments made about the size of a baby's head posing a problem when moving past the pelvis and vaginal outlet. These have also caused an unwarranted fear surrounding birth in the minds of women.

Actually, it is very rare that a mother will carry and birth a child whose head is too large to make the birth journey. It can happen, but not often. Relax and release these fear-provoking thoughts. Here's how it all happens.

This news about fontanels is probably the best news that a pregnant mother can receive. Most people know about the "soft spot" that is evident on a newly born baby's head. Not commonly known is that the soft spot is not there to accommodate the growth of the baby's skull as she gets older. It is there to accommodate her smooth, easy descent through the birth path and her emergence. The process is appropriately called "moulding." The sutures of the baby's skull mould to the contours of your birth path, and they facilitate the turns that the baby makes as she descends.

Surrounding the bony frame of the baby's skull at the top and back of her head is a flexible membranous material called fontanels. This material, much like the texture of a heavy canvas fabric, allows the bones of the skull to "mould" and overlap each other. The usual procedure of the bones involves the lower back suture moving up and under the upper back sutures. Likewise, the front sutures move up and under the front of the upper sutures. All of this reduces the circumference of the baby's head. As the baby emerges, most often the overlapped top sutures can be seen briefly, but as the baby emerges fully, they move back into their normal positioning, leaving what is commonly called the "soft spot." Until the skull suture fully closes, which in some cases can take well over a year for the frontal suture, the soft spot is protected by the membranous fontanels.

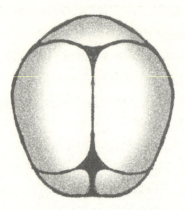

Bone Formation of Baby's Skull (Top View)

Natural Expulsive Reflex (NER)

When the baby is ready for his gradual descent to crowning and birth, your body's natural expulsive reflex (NER) will rhythmically move the baby down with natural pulsations, as you assist with soft gentle Birth Breathing during a surge. You may be aware of the downward motion of the baby, and you will feel a full, bulging feeling at your perineum when the baby is crowning.

You remain in a comfortable, relaxed state and just gently breathe your baby down as you've practised. There is no need for forced pushing.

On this subject, Dr. White further says:

> *"She feels the progress of the baby's moving, and she becomes more satisfied that she is accomplishing something.*
>
> *At this point, the mother may desire to help by bearing down and she should be allowed to, but (if there is no cause for concern) she should not be urged to do so. She should begin this work only when she feels she must, not because she or the attendant thinks it is a good idea. (Most babies do not require urgent pushing, though attendants may strongly encourage such activities because they do not trust the body's ability to expel the baby naturally.)"*

This natural function of your body will assist in clearing your baby's lungs of mucous and may avoid the use of a suction bulb, which is a rude welcome afforded your baby, especially when suctioning is done on the rim of the perineum before your baby is fully born. The benefits and importance of the natural expulsive reflex cannot be over emphasised. When you avoid forced pushing, you maintain a flow of oxygen to your baby and avoid the foetal distress that often occurs in that late state of birthing. Your baby maintains a healthy heart rate. Both baby and mother birth without severe pain, though you may be aware of a bit of pressure. There is no physiological reason for forced pushing. As explained earlier, this is a conditioning that occurred when women were taught to birth. There should be no pain if you use calm breathing to avoid a spasm-like breath and don't force the baby against tissues that may not be ready to receive him.

Let's take a look at the pros and cons of both of the breathing styles used during the actual descent and birth of the baby.

Mother-Directed Birth Breathing	Staff-Directed Forced Pushing
Allows parents to maintain control over their birthing	Tires mother and reduces her effectiveness and participation in birthing experience
Conserves mother's energy	Closes and constricts vaginal passage ahead of baby
Provides continual supply of oxygen to the baby	Emergency intervention can result.
	Mother becomes exhausted; baby is distressed
Gently opens the birth path for smooth descent	Ruptures eye and facial blood vessels
Increases prospect of birthing over an intact perineum	Limits flow of oxygen to baby, often causing heart-rate deceleration
Perineal tissues unfold naturally for the gentle emergence of baby	Surrenders control of birthing to others
Baby maintains healthy heart rate during descent	Contributes to tearing or the need for episiotomy

On occasion, staff members may tell you that breathing down works for a while, but you need to switch to forced pushing at the end of the descent. If you are using the Power of Nothing, it will just be time that you are not expending a strong effort and you won't be exhausted. Many women find that it is actually faster. Birthing in water will add to your relaxation and to the suppleness of your perineum. You need to trust your natural expulsive reflex to do its job. Sometimes staff members become a bit impatient, but if you stick to your natural expulsive reflex you'll find that it will help your baby to emerge in less time and with less risk of distress. To optimise this gift, you will want to practise Birth Breathing daily on the toilet as you expel a bowel movement. The same expulsive muscle action is used in both situations. (See the section on Breathing Techniques)

Perineal Folds

Because the perineum is toned, the rim is supple and gently unfolds as the baby passes down and out of the vaginal outlet. You will feel some pressure as this happens, but pressure has its own numbing effect. We experience this happening when resting on an arm or a hand while sleeping or when we cross our legs for any length of time. So will the rim of the perineum numb when the baby passes through it. You will not have to deal with the myth of the burning ring, and most mothers don't need an episiotomy. This same pressure will kindly numb the area should you have a small tear.

As the baby emerges from the vaginal outlet past the rim of perineum, you will not experience the stretching of the perineum that most people speak of. The folds of the perineum will gently open. All of the folds are there, and they do not require the assistance of an attendant to pull or tug by "ironing the perineum," as it is sometimes called.

The fact that you will not be forcefully pushing your baby also enhances the gradual unfolding of the rim. It works. Just as the anal rim unfolds, so do the folds of the perineum. It does not need the assistance of a staff member if you have prepared with the perineal massage.

Umbilical Pulsations

When the baby is born, the cord is left unclamped and intact for optimum benefit to the baby. When the cord is left unclamped, the baby's blood supply continues to provide him with oxygen while he gradually becomes accustomed to breathing on his own. This is a very important adjustment that your baby is making, and he needs to be accommodated in this way. By allowing the baby to use his own blood, there is no sudden, sometimes painful, gasp for air. It is also not necessary for attendants to vigorously rub or poke or prod to start the baby breathing or urging him to cry, all of which create an abrupt and confusing experience for the baby. The placental blood remains to oxygenate the baby until his lungs are fully functioning. Umbilical pulsations also allow the baby to receive the blood that is rightfully his to increase his iron storage and ward off anaemia. The placenta will detach more easily when allowed to empty naturally.

There is no particular risk to a baby being born with the cord around its neck, contrary to all the drama that is used to describe this condition. More than a third of babies are born with the cord situated around their necks. The only true danger is when the cord is wrapped and compressed so that circulation is cut off.

Most care providers gently remove the cord by slipping it over the baby's neck at the time of emergence, and the baby continues to be born without incident.

Placental Release

After your baby is born, the cord will continue to pulse until the optimum amount of blood is returned to the baby. The baby will instinctually feel the need to crawl to your nipple for his first feeding. This should be allowed. The scent of colostrum will lure the baby to your nipple and set him in the right direction. This is in keeping with the instinct of all mammals. When the baby is sucking, more oxytocin is released, and this helps to release your placenta from the uterine wall. It also provides you with even more of that valuable "love hormone" that helps to make the mother-baby connection. It helps to allay your baby's fears and gives him a sense of security and safety. It makes the birth afterglow that much more special as you and your partner bond with the baby.

It is important that you learn the importance and significance of these perks of nature so that you can learn to trust that birthing is, indeed, intended to be natural and accomplished with ease.

Relaxation Routine

Muscles send messages to each other.
Clenched fists, a tight mouth, a furrowed brow,
all send signals to the birth-passage muscles, the very
ones that need to be loosened. Opening up to relax
these upper-body parts relaxes the lower ones.

William Sears and Martha Sears, *The Birth Book*

M ost athletes will readily advise that relaxation and visualisation are crucial to successful performance. Golfers quickly
learn not to "press," but to release and let go. It is not uncommon to see Olympic athletes standing off to the side running visualisations of their perfect performance through their minds. Sports greats
know that stress and tension in the mind equate to stress and tension
in the body; the two cannot be separated. Conquering stress and fear
is what allows sports figures to appear to perform so effortlessly. It's
impressive.

There are six basic techniques that we will cover in this section.
Each technique has several alternatives so you can choose the one (or

more) that you find most effective and that you like best. Learning to use all six techniques so that they become second nature to you will prepare your body and mind for the birth process.

The Six Basic HypnoBirthing Component Techniques

Education	**Relaxation**
Breathing	**Visualisation**
Deepening	**Affirmations**

Taking the time to practise these techniques is an essential part of your daily routine. There is absolutely no substitute for the work you will do to condition your mind and body in preparation for birth. You cannot simply attend classes and hope that the conditioning will occur without your dedication to making it happen. Conditioning involves your mind and your body. A skier would never attempt to compete in a tournament unless his body was conditioned. A runner would never attempt to enter a marathon unless his body was conditioned.

While birthing should not be the exhausting, pushing-your-body-to-the-edge feat that athletes face, it nevertheless requires the same kind of discipline so that when the time comes, you are ready. Since you are conditioning your mind for ultimate relaxation, it is important that you form a pattern that your mind can automatically respond to when it comes time for your birthing. It is time well spent, and it can cut the time and the effort you will spend in your labour. As one who has been there, I can emphatically say that conditioning is a must. You can't slough it off and hope that you'll get lucky.

Your Relaxation Programme

By far one of the most effective ways of dealing with tension, stress, and discomfort without drugs is your own conditioned ability to slip into relaxation and visualisation quickly and at any given moment. In HypnoBirthing you will learn relaxation techniques and visualisations that will see you through your labour and quickly bring about a renewed state of energy following your birthing. It is important that you rehearse these techniques so that you can call them up readily when they are needed.

Establishing Your Routine

- When planning your relaxation, select a time when you won't be disturbed. Take the receiver off the phone or turn off the ringer and answering machine.

- Set aside the same time each day and dedicate yourself to that time.

- Choose a comfortable practice spot that has soft, dim light and make that the place you will use daily.

- Be sure that your bladder is empty.

- Warmth is essential to relieve tension so use a soft throw over your body. Wear clothes that are soft and not binding.

- Use HypnoBirthing CDs or MP3s. We recommend Stephen Halpern's *Comfort Zone* for consistency, as that is the background music used for the Rainbow Relaxation. This music contains tones and rhythms that the body responds to best.

Positions for Relaxation

Your body is the best source of information for the position you will assume when doing relaxation. The general rule is to use the position in which you feel most comfortable. The two recommended positions to follow are Nesting and Side Lying.

Early in your pregnancy, you will no doubt be comfortable on your back while you practise relaxation. Later in your pregnancy, you will want to elevate your upper body to accommodate the extra weight of the baby. Once you gain more weight, you may choose to use a different position. Avoid lying flat on your back, to ensure that the pressure from your growing baby does not obstruct the inferior vena cava, which is a main source of blood and oxygen to your baby.

Nesting

Nesting is one of the best ways of reaching a fully relaxed state quickly. To make your relaxation nest:

- Place one or two pillows under your head and shoulders.

- Allow your shoulders to drift downward and outward.

- Place one pillow under each arm. Allow your arms to gently rest on top of your side pillows with your elbows slightly bent.

- Fingers should be gently and softly cupped.

- Place pillows under the bend of each knee.

- Feet should be about six inches apart, turned outward, relaxed.

Lateral Position

The lateral position is chosen most often by birthing mothers during late labour and frequently for birthing their babies. It is also a position that is usually assumed for sleeping during pregnancy.

- Lie on your left side with the left shoulder, neck, and left side of the head resting on a pillow. The left arm should be placed loosely by your left side.

- With the elbow bent, rest the right arm to the side of the pillow.

- The left leg should be straight down, with the knee slightly bent.

- Bend the right leg up, placing the knee even with your abdomen, with one or two pillows under the knee for support.

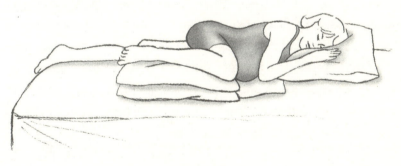

Lateral Position

As you continue to work with the exercises for relaxation, you'll find that each one gives you an explanation of the benefits of the exercise and a brief script that you can use in practise with your birth companion. As you practise these recommended exercises, you will naturally find the one or ones that feel most comfortable for you. It is not necessary that you work with all of them. It is more important that you work with the technique that works best for you.

Facial Relaxation

Achieving deep facial relaxation is most important, as it will set the tone for the rest of your body. The lower jaw area directly affects the vaginal opening. When your lower jaw is relaxed, the vaginal area will be relaxed also. Relax your mouth, just where your teeth meet your pallet. This will prevent your upper and lower teeth from becoming clenched. When you have mastered the art of facial relaxation, your jaws will be totally relaxed, with the lower jaw slightly receded. You will be able to bring yourself into a natural state of relaxation instantly.

Facial Relaxation Technique

Let your eyelids slowly close. Don't try to force them shut. Just let them gently meet. Place your awareness on the muscles in and around your eyes. As you feel a natural drooping of the eye muscles, sense relaxation spreading from your forehead, down across your eyelids, over your cheekbones and around your jaws. Let your lower jaw recede as your teeth part. Your eyelids will feel heavier as your cheeks and your jaw go limp. Bring the relaxation within your eyes to a level where it seems as though your eyelids just refuse to work. Place the tip of your tongue at your palate where your upper teeth and palate meet, bringing about a sense of peace and well-being as you connect with an energy orbit in your body. Feel your head making a dent into your pillow. As you practise this technique, you will feel your neck, shoulders, and elbows droop. Picture your shoulders opening outward and sinking down into the frame of your body as you go deeply into relaxation.

Relaxation Techniques

Once you have learned to bring your breathing into a smooth, rhythmic pace and you can ease yourself into relaxation effortlessly, you can then learn to bring your relaxation on instantly by using one of the methods included here. You do not need to master all of these techniques. You will naturally turn to the ones that are most effective for you and that you like best.

Progressive Relaxation

Sitting in a comfortable chair or sofa, associate each of the designated parts of your body from the top of your head to your toes with the number that corresponds to it on the illustration that follows. Take a deep breath, then as you exhale let it all instantly flow down through your body, causing your muscles to go totally limp. We refer to this state as "Lucy Limp" (Loosey Limp), the name of a soft doll that is like a Beanie Baby.

Eventually, you will be able to take one deep breath and rapidly count off the numbers as you exhale, bringing those parts of your body immediately into a limp state. The more rapidly you think the numbers, the more rapidly you will feel the effects. In using this practise, you should let your body go absolutely limp from the top of your head down to your toes. Let your head hang loose and forward, and let your arms and hands fall limp down by your side.

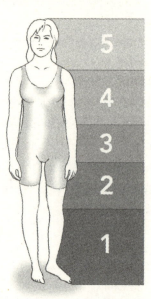

Disappearing Letters

A similar technique for bringing yourself into a deep level of relaxation is to use the Disappearing Letters exercise. It is perhaps the easiest of all the instant relaxation techniques that you will use. It is especially helpful if you feel stressed during the day at work or home or if you need some help falling asleep. When using this technique as an aid to falling asleep, you will actually feel your head creating a deeper indentation into your pillow as your neck muscles thoroughly relax.

With practice, you will find that by the time you reach the first or second "C," the rest of the letters of the alphabet will be erased from your mind. It will be too much effort to say or think the letters, and your body will be limp, as described earlier. This exercise is one of the fastest ways to bring yourself into a wonderful, comfortable state at any time. I recommend it especially to maintain a feeling of calm during that period of adjustment after your baby is born.

Disappearing Letters Technique

- Close your eyes.

- Take in a quick, deep breath—pause.

- Quickly visualise the letters rolling by or coming forward and mentally say to yourself quickly while you exhale:

   AAA—BBB—CCC—D . . . etc.

- Allow your head, neck, shoulders, and upper torso to instantly sink into the frame of your body. Give yourself permission to let your arms, hands, and legs hang loosely. This can be accomplished in seconds and will be very useful for you when you are birthing, as well as at other times.

Light Touch Massage

Birth companions are taught the art of applying Light Touch Massage, a technique developed by Constance Palinsky of Michigan after much research into pain management and the release of endorphins.

The theory of Light Touch is that the smooth muscle just below the surface of the skin, called erector pili, reacts by contracting when stimulated. When this occurs, the muscle pulls up the surface hair, which becomes erect and causes goose bumps. The goose bumps, in turn, help to create endorphins, those feel-good hormones that promote relaxation.

We use Light Touch Massage in birthing because when endorphins are secreted, catecholamine is not. The two cannot co-exist. So the goal of relaxation is to create the feel-good endorphins so that catecholamines cannot take hold. The technique is very simple, yet effective. It is a wonderful comfort measure that the birthing companion brings to the labour room and as a means of nurturing during pregnancy. It is a great way for couples to feel physically closer to each other in the later stages of pregnancy.

The creation of endorphins resulting from practising Light Touch Massage helps to keep our mums calm and comfortable, both prior to birthing and while in labour. If, while the birth companion is applying Light Touch, he extends his hands out and around the sides of the breasts and nipples to apply light nipple stimulation, not only are endorphins produced, but also the hormone oxytocin is created, which naturally enhances uterine surges. For that reason, until you are approaching the very end of your term, the birth companion should not massage the nipples when practising this technique.

Light Touch Massage can be applied while the mother is sitting on a birth ball leaning on pillows at the side of a bed. If the couple is in a hospital, they can request that the foot of the bed be adjusted to create a kneeler. Mothers can also have the head of the bed adjusted upright so that she can kneel on the centre of the bed and rest her arms and head at the top of the bed on a pillow. This is an excellent position to give her the advantage of being upright when baby is descending during birth. If birthing is taking place at home or in a birthing centre, the same effect can be achieved by kneeling on a pillow in front of a chair, a sofa, or at the side of a bed with pillows stacked upright for you to rest your arms and head on. Your birthing companion can kneel behind you while administering Light Touch Massage as illustrated or can also use a chair.

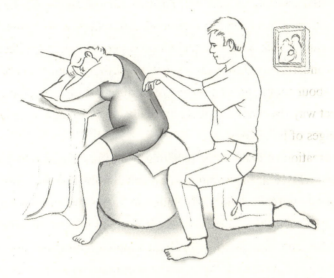

Birth Companion Applies Light Touch Massage

While children, as well as adults, enjoy Light Touch Massage, it should not be used with infants as their nervous system is not developed sufficiently to be able to experience the kind of stimulation that Light Tough offers. After three or four months, you can use Light Touch to calm a fretful child.

Light Touch Massage Technique

- The birth companion places the BACK side of his or her fingers so that they meet at the base of the tailbone. The fingers are then drawn up and out from the spine in a V-like motion. The pattern is gradually continued upward across the back until the base of the neck is reached. The hands are then brought around the neck and to the sides of the ears. The undersides of the arms and around the elbows are particularly effective areas for the massage.

- The second motion involves placing the BACK of the fingers at the base of the spine and then, as before, gradually working upward, forming a horizontal, figure-eight pattern that criss-crosses at the centre of the back.

- This technique is demonstrated in HypnoBirthing classes, and you will have the opportunity to practise it as well. It is an extremely important element in HypnoBirthing. When the birth companion does it right, the mother will be amazed at the results.

Anchors

In the practice of hypnosis, an anchor is a means of creating a lasting imprint or signal through an association with a gesture, sound, image, or touch. The thought or suggestion is said to be anchored into the memory of the subconscious. In HypnoBirthing, the birth companion will plant an anchor that is a signal to you to go more deeply into relaxation by placing his hand on your shoulder during your practise sessions. The birth companion instructs the mother that when she feels the hand being placed on her shoulder, with a gentle downward press, she will immediately relax twice as deeply as she is at the moment. You will be amazed at the power of this technique. I suggest that you make it a regular part of your practice together.

Anchors can be used in any number of ways for birthing and in other situations. One woman in a HypnoBirthing class kept forgetting to take her vitamins. She anchored a reminder that when she picked up her car keys to leave in the morning, she would remember to take her vitamins. She never missed a day after that.

Breathing Techniques

There are only three gentle breathing techniques used in Hypno-Birthing: Calm Breathing, Surge Breathing, and Birth Breathing.

Calm Breathing

Calm Breathing is simply what its name implies. This breath can easily be applied on a regular basis to many situations in your life when you are feeling tense, frightened, or fatigued. It is a breathing style designed to help you enter a calm, relaxed state so that you can continue with imagery and visualisation practice. You'll find it especially helpful after your baby is born when you just sit quietly with your baby and connect with her. It is the breath usually used at the beginning of a meditation or relaxation session.

Calm breathing maintains the sufficient, continual supply of oxygen to your baby during labour. This oxygen is the most important fuel for the working muscles in the uterus. That is why proper breathing is so important to your relaxation. The Calm Breathing technique is used at

actice to help your body gradually

axation. You will want to focus your

y in your programme.

u to achieve relaxation when you are

birth companion. It is also one of the

ie relaxation between uterine surges dur-

ing birth............ will help you to conserve energy during the thinning and opening ....ase of labour. To establish a proper breathing technique for Calm Breathing, practise the following exercise.

Calm Breathing Technique

- Relax and settle into the comfort of a chair or sofa and let pillows support your head and neck.

- Allow your head to gently lean forward toward your chest, or let it rest back onto pillows behind you.

- Let your eyelids gently meet without forcing them shut.

- Your mouth should be softly closed with your lips touching lightly.

- Place the tip of your tongue at your palate where your teeth and your palate meet and feel the wonderful sense of relaxation drifting throughout your body.

- Take in a short breath through your nose, to a count of four: mentally recite "In–2–3–4" on the intake. Feel your stomach rise as you draw the breath up and into the back of your throat. Pause.

- As you exhale, mentally recite "Out–2–3–4–5–6–7–8." Do not exhale through your mouth. As you breathe out very slowly through your nose, direct the energy of the breath down and inward toward the back of your throat, allowing your shoulders to droop into the frame of your body. Breathe your body down into relaxation. Release all tension and let go.

To determine if you are doing this exercise correctly, place your left hand on your stomach and your right hand on the lower part of your chest. As you inhale, you should feel your left hand rising as though your stomach were inflating like a balloon. As you exhale, you will feel your hands fold into each other as your chest and stomach create a crevice.

Calm Breathing is easy to master. You will use it regularly in your classes and in your home practice. You'll feel relaxation coming more easily and rapidly each time you do it. When you have mastered the concept, it will not be necessary for you to recite numbers or test with your hands to guide yourself into this state. After doing this only a few times, you will be able to bring your body into a deep state of relaxation in preparation for further deepening work.

Surge Breathing

The name of this breathing, Surge Breathing, suggests when it is used in labour. This breathing style is used throughout the entire period that your cervix is opening and thinning. Each time that you experience a uterine surge or wave, this breath helps you to work with your birthing body. It is actually assisting labour progress rather than resisting. It works in conjunction with the vertical muscles as they draw up the horizontal muscles to allow the cervix to open. HypnoBirthing mothers find that because of this feature, their surges last a shorter time than usual, and, therefore, the opening and thinning phase is shortened.

You will want to devote time to Surge Breathing, as it is this technique that will be with you until it is time to breathe your baby down to crowning.

The following exercise will take you through the steps of Surge Breathing.

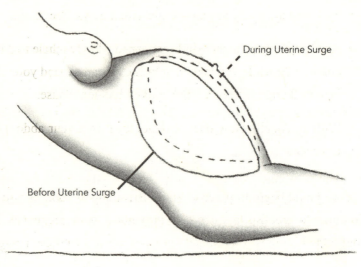

During Uterine Surge

Before Uterine Surge

The Uterus During Surge

Surge Breathing Technique

- In a lateral position, place a pillow under your back and shoulders.

- Place both hands across the top of your abdomen with your fingers loosely meshed between each other.

- Breathe down into your abdomen to clear your breath.

- Using only your abdominal muscles, take in a breath and let your abdomen expand into your cupped fingers. Do this several times and note the way your abdomen moves outward as it expands. Once more, expand the abdomen and note the motion and the way in which your fingers move outward. Repeat this several times to get the feeling of the expanding and receding abdomen.

- Now you are ready to practise the actual Surge Breathing.

- Again with your fingers slightly cupped, slowly inhale to a rapid count of 20 while you take in your breath and expand your abdomen as though it were a large colored balloon. Pause.

- With an equally slow pace, exhale down into your abdomen as it recedes.

You should begin to practise Surge Breathing as soon as you can. Continue to practise this exercise throughout your pregnancy until your body becomes conditioned to this expansion with each surge.

Birth Breathing

The third style of breathing is called Birth Breathing. It's the technique that you will use during birthing when you are breathing your baby down through the birth path to emergence during the birthing phase. You will begin to practise Birth Breathing immediately.

Like the other two breathing styles, Birth Breathing clearly describes when this breath is applied. Once your cervix has reached a degree of opening sufficient for the baby to pass down out of the cervix, Birth

Breathing will step in and will assist the natural expulsive reflex (NER) of your body to move your baby down to crowning and birth.

Birth Breathing. . . Don't Push Me, Mummy

Birth Breathing is used when you are breathing your baby down during the birthing phase of labour. It is intended to assist the natural expulsive reflex (NER) of your body to move your baby gently down to crowning and birth.

Birth Breathing is NOT pushing. Pushing can be counterproductive and actually slow down the birthing process. The concept of pushing your baby out is a rude and unnecessary one. This is one of the classic examples of how women, contrary to their natural birthing instincts, have been taught how to birth.

For hundreds of years, totally anaesthetised women had their babies extracted from their bodies with forceps. They were unable to immediately see their babies and sometimes did not see or hold their babies until the following day. As a result of this extraction and the other unnecessary procedures that resulted, women were confined to their beds for days following their births.

Few doctors had the opportunity to witness a baby being naturally born, as most natural births were still taking place at home with midwives.

Unanaesthetised birth came upon the birthing scene when Dr. Ferdinand Lamaze introduced his concept of easier birthing through focused attention that distracted mothers from the pain of birthing. The problem presented, however, was that so many birth professionals, accustomed only to seeing women giving birth with forceps, did not believe that the baby would descend and emerge on his own. (A belief that remains even today as HypnoBirthing mothers are told that their babies will not be born unless the mother is willing "to help yourself and push that baby out.")

It was then thought, however, that since there was no means of extracting the baby with instruments, the baby would have to be "pushed" down through the birth path and out past the vaginal outlet.

A technique was devised and readily accepted in birthing circles. Staff members "coached" the birthing mother in unison, while she held her breath and violently pushed, usually to the count of 10. They cheered her on while one staff member and a birth companion would draw her knees up to her shoulders with each surge. Another means was lifting the mother's head and shoulders forward, forming what was called a "C position," while other staff members counted 1 and 2 and 3, all the way up to 10. Because the mother's pushing caused the blood vessels in her face and eyes to bulge and become purple from the violent pushing, this was called "purple pushing."

Sadly, today this very scene still plays out in most hospital births. It has become the source of many attempts at humour. No one seems to question the indignity that the mother experiences during this time.

Forced pushing creates stress for the birthing mother, which is self-defeating in that it closes the sphincters of the vagina ahead of the descending baby. Any woman who attempts to simulate forced pushing will immediately verify that there is a tensing of the muscles in the lower birth path, not a release.

In spite of this, most birth professionals cling to the loud, chaotic means of "helping" the baby out.

There has been much written about the inefficiency of forced pushing and the possible damaging effect it has on the muscles of the birthing woman's pelvic floor.

While the woman who finds herself unable to push because she has been administered an epidural is allowed to "labour down" by letting her body naturally expel her baby, the woman in the next room who has deliberately planned for a natural birth is expected to forcefully "push her baby out." It is an unnecessary carry over, when we consider that women in comas have given birth undetected.

With Birth Breathing, there is no need for a lengthy period of hard, violent pushing during descent. Your baby's descent will be gradual, but it will not necessarily take longer. The natural pulsations of your body will move your baby down the birth path efficiently and gently. Many mothers report using only two or three Birth Breaths to bring their babies to full emergence. That's because the sphincters at the outlet are not tense and closed. The relaxed body will naturally open for you. Birth Breathing also gives your baby the advantage of a kinder, safer, and gentler birth.

Forced pushing can exhaust you and press your baby against a resistant passage that is not yet receptive to his journey. Stories of exhaustive pushing that extends over hours bear out the fact that the baby will descend when he and the birth path are ready. There is no need to rush. The natural birthing process has a purpose that must be respected and trusted.

Often women themselves will speak of an overwhelming urge to push taking over. If this is felt, it is also because of conditioning that stems from a deeply embedded notion that babies cannot descend on their own. We seem to be the only mammals who turn our birthings into what appears to be a gymnastic event, complete with "squat bars" and knotted ropes on which mothers can suspend themselves. This scene hardly holds a mirror up to nature. Our animal sisters elect to gently expel their babies.

A calm, gentle nudging bre[...]
lishing the same kind of rela[...]
Breathing practice. Even if you[...]
to push," surrendering to this im[...]
around, as it limits the amount of o[...]
cause concern on the part of caregiv[...]
decelerate. It may lead to the very s[...]
worked so hard to avoid. Let your bab[...] ......ne the
pace. Breathe down into your body to n[...] .aginal outlet and follow whatever lead your baby takes.

Birth Breathing is one of the most important of all the exercises you
will practise. It is easily accomplished by using your body's natural
expulsive reflex that occurs each and every time you use the toilet to
expel your daily stool. It is the most natural function that the expulsive
muscles use routinely.

When your cervix has reached completion, you should feel the urge
now to breathe downward rather than upward. This will be a natural
transition for you. Rather than allow your body to slip in a spasm-like
surge, you will remain in whatever position is comfortable for you and
simply allow Calm Breaths to guide you into breathing down.

Birth Breathing Technique

- Assume a comfortable position.

- Your body will feel the urge to breathe down, and you should
  only breathe down when in surge.

- Follow the lead of your body and your baby.

- Your mouth should be softly closed and not pursed; no breath
  should escape through the mouth.

in and let out through the nose.

remain in an amnesiac state as you and baby birth
ther.

- Use Calm Breathing to avoid pushing.

- Direct the energy of your breath to the lower back of your throat
  and allow that thrust of energy to move down through your back
  as it gently nudges your baby down and out through your vaginal
  outlet.

- Inhale again and direct that energy to the back of your throat and
  down your back all the way to the vaginal outlet.

- Keep the vaginal outlet and your anal passage open in between
  breaths so you will not lose the momentum.

The perfect place to practise this exercise is on the toilet as you are
guiding the stool down and out of the anal passage. Make it a point to
do this each and every time you are using the toilet in this way. You
will find that you will accomplish the task easier and more quickly
each time.

Visualisation Techniques

The breathing and relaxation exercises in the previous chapters are fundamental elements of HypnoBirthing and should be practised daily. The visualisation exercises are merely tools to help you during labour. You may find one or all of them useful to calm your mind and relax your body. Therefore, you should experiment to find the ones you like. These visualisation exercises, while helpful, do not need to be part of your daily routine. The exception is Rainbow Relaxation.

Rainbow Relaxation

Rainbow Relaxation is the cornerstone of our relaxation and visualisation programme. It incorporates the many colors that are associated with the energy centres of our body. The background music, "The Comfort Zone," is a composition by Steven Halpern, a world-renowned author, composer, and recording artist whose sounds are designed to bring your thoughts into harmony with the natural flow of energy within your body.

The following explanation of how the Rainbow Relaxation technique is used will give you an understanding of what to expect and how the important repeated practise with this recording is more effective than a scripted theme in effecting your ultimate conditioning for birthing. You should practise the entire Rainbow Relaxation every day. Your HypnoBirthing practitioner will provide you with the Rainbow Relaxation recording along with your textbook, both of which are included in your tuition.

During deep relaxation practice, the brain and the nervous system become saturated with the picture of your specific goals or ideals. The repetition of these images seems so real to the subconscious that the images become imprinted in your mind and embedded in your subconscious. The assimilation of these visions creates acceptance, belief, and confidence in achieving the desired outcome. In your case these images are easier, gentler birthing and a calm, peaceful life.

If there are any words or images on the CD that you don't feel comfortable with, just mentally substitute a word or a phrase that you feel better suits you and let that substitution bring you even deeper into relaxation. All hypnosis is self-hypnosis, and it's important to know that no one else brings you into this state except yourself. Hypnosis is a therapy of consent. If you are finding that you need help in reaching a deep level of relaxation, speak to your practitioner so that together you can get to the root of why this is happening.

Often mums will question if the time they are spending in practice is working for them. They find that after one or two practise sessions, they no longer are able to stay with the material because they drift off into their own thoughts or they fall into a deep sleep. Actually, nothing could be better. If this should happen to you, be aware that you are not actually asleep. You have successfully conditioned your mind to respond immediately by bringing yourself into a state that seems like sleep. If this happens regularly, just know that your subconscious is tuned in to your practise sessions and is processing them for you. That is part of the conditioning effect.

For the purpose of conditioning your mind to relax, Rainbow Relaxation does not have a sequence or "story" to it. The repetition of the wording is especially designed to help you tune out your surroundings and bring you to the level of relaxation that you want to reach quickly. As pleasant as it may be, visualising scenes in nature or spending an inordinate amount of time in progressive relaxation during your practice sessions is not necessary. Whether you mentally visualise the process, your birthing companion walks you through it, or you listen to the CD, you will easily master the art after the first week if you allow yourself to just go with it. If you are enjoying the process, you may obtain other discs from the Institute, but the Rainbow exercise will do the trick for you if you are conditioning your mind and body to respond with deep relaxation.

The birth companion is an active participant throughout the birthing experience. Rather than an onlooker who vacillates between feeling helpless and unknowledgeable, in HypnoBirthing the birth companion is actually the trained facilitator and primary support person for the birthing mother. The perinatal bonding that takes place among mother, baby, and the birthing companion during this wonderful interlude, combined with the mother's conditioned relaxation, is the whole key to achieving a satisfying birth for all of you. The baby becomes familiar with the birth companion's voice during these sessions, and all of this contributes to the important post-natal bonding and helps the newborn's adjustment.

As often as possible, the birthing companion should practise the Rainbow Relaxation with you, following the outline below. This practice is important so that you will be able to drift into a deep level of relaxation on hearing your birth companion's voice. When you practise with your birth companion, it is better to keep your sessions shorter, but more frequent. This will prevent your time together from becoming a lengthy chore that can be put off until you "can find more time."

While reciting the sequence of colours, the birth companion should stroke your hand and arm in a soft downward motion, simulating the flow of natural relaxation that will drift throughout your body while you are in the thinning and opening phase of labour.

The Birth Companion's Reading (to follow) provides a visualisation of moving through labour that can help you to envision a smooth, calm birth. This can be practised alternately with the Rainbow Relaxation. When you choose to use the Birth Companion's Reading, have the mother picture herself stepping into the happy scene of both of you holding and bonding with your baby seconds after birth. This is an important visualisation for creating an imprint of a positive, happy outcome.

The practice that you do together is intended to strengthen the conditioning that comes from your learning to respond to your birth companion's voice and touch. It will also strengthen the bond between you as you anticipate your upcoming birthing.

Rainbow Relaxation Technique

- Find a place where you both can be comfortable and where the lighting is soft. Mother should be sitting in a chair with her head resting on the back of the chair or on a sofa with pillows beneath her head and shoulders so that the top of her body is elevated slightly.

- Mother, gently bring yourself into a deep state of relaxation—the kind you have been teaching yourself. Breathe in relaxation and breathe down relaxation throughout your body, using the Calm Breathing technique.

- Once you have brought yourself into this calm state of relaxation, picture yourself gently resting on a bed of strawberry-coloured mist that is about a foot and a half high. Picture the soft red mist as a mist of natural relaxation flowing through and around your body. Continue to relax until it seems that your body is almost weightless and seems to meld into the mist. Feel the coloured mist caressing your shoulders, midriff, buttocks, and legs. Allow yourself to "let go" and feel as though you are floating on the strawberry-coloured mist. Feel the gentle sway. See this soft mist saturating your body as you go deeper into relaxation. Feel your body growing numb, almost as though it were a piece of soft, strawberry-coloured cloth. Allow yourself to feel the mist of deep relaxation permeating your mind and body from the top of your head to your toes. Feel the tingling of relaxation on the soles of your feet. Imagine your own natural mist of relaxation swirling over and around your body—mind and body at peace and tranquil.

- Now picture yourself resting on a bed of pale, orange-coloured mist, while your body becomes even more comfortable. Follow the same visualisation as you did for the soft strawberry colour. Imagine the coloured mist sweeping across your body, starting at the top of your head, caressing your shoulders, chest, arms, and legs, and slowly drifting all the way down to your feet. Again, feel the tingling of relaxation on the soles of your feet and know that you are going deeper in relaxation.

- Next picture yourself on a mist of soft yellow, with the coloured mist surrounding your body, starting at the very top of your head and drifting down across your cheeks, jaws, and mouth. Now the same quality of relaxation slips down across your shoulders, upper arms, elbows, and hands and wanders down through your abdomen, legs, and to the very bottom of the soles of your feet.

- Continue the visualisation until all the remaining colours of the rainbow have been envisioned—green, blue, and indigo, then white for clarity.

- Now slowly bring yourself back to the room, feeling alert and energised.

The Birth Companion's Reading

The Birth Companion reading can be alternative to the Rainbow. This reading is adapted from one originally composed by Henry Leo Bolduc for his wife Joan when they were preparing for the birth of their baby. The script appears in Henry's book *Self-Hypnosis: Creating Your Own Destiny*.

His reading was an outpouring of the awe with which a father views this wonderful miracle. Henry expresses sensitivity to perinatal bonding when he points out that the attitude and philosophy of the mother and the birth companion are as much a gentle suggestion for the child during birthing as it is reassurance for the mother.

Thanks to Henry for allowing me to incorporate a few HypnoBirthing images into his script.

New life is forming, growing and moving within you. You are part of the promise and the destiny of life itself. A very important event is taking place in your life . . . a wonderfully normal, natural, biological, and spiritual event. You're going to have a baby. What is happening now is the process of birthing and freeing the kicking, moving little being who's been a part of your body for so long.

Soon it will be time for the baby to become its own separate person. One cycle is ending and, immediately, another is beginning. What has been called "labour" is that in-between experience . . . the fulcrum . . . that small, short period of time and space between the baby's two worlds.

Change from one stage to another brings pressure, and then release. You will soon experience this as the change is completed and fulfilled. You can feel this and embrace it and welcome it as refreshing and totally natural.

With mind, you build a healthy attitude and happy expectation. Happy childbirth has much to do with a healthy, joyous, loving anticipation. It is something remarkably beautiful. Being a channel of new life is said to be a spiritual experience. With this understanding, total relaxation, and serene breathing, all discomfort is lessened and often entirely absent.

As you begin labour, meditate on the tremendous universal force . . . the life force of nature with which you are in complete harmony during this experience.

Whenever you feel your body begin to surge, actively think "release" and "let go" of tension. There is a time for experiencing that uterine wave, flowing with it, and ultimately releasing and letting go.

g *to relax, to flow and melt with the very rhythm of*
axation *and positive expectation, you have come to*
gs *are possible.*

In your mind's eye, picture the shore of a lake or an ocean. Watch the endless waves softly brushing to the shore . . . the ebb and flow of the water. Observe it advancing and withdrawing over the sand. Become a part of it, flowing into it. Become a part of the rhythm of the waves within your own body . . . the surge and release.

Breathe in the natural relaxants of your own body . . . endorphins, many times more effective than the strongest drugs known to man . . . create your own serenity and release it throughout your body . . . breathing in and breathing through . . . giving birth to your baby.

With proper physical, spiritual, and mental exercise, you are preparing yourself for this wonderful celebration of life. As you get into the rhythm and work with your mind and body, the easier and smoother it becomes. Each time you hear your birth companion's voice and feel the gentle touch: the more easily your relaxation deepens.

Breathe . . . slowly, confidently, gently. Each time you breathe in, breathe in relaxation and peace. Each time you breathe out, breathe out stress, as the body's natural endorphins willfully breathe out tension and stress.

Feel only the sway of the wave that is bringing your baby closer and closer to birth. Relax and flow with your body's natural rhythm, confident in the fact that your body knows what to do. Give your birthing over to your body. Trust it. Relax and let it do its job.

With your mind's eye and your inner senses, mentally and emotionally feel yourself joyfully, totally aware and participating. See it as already accomplished. Listen with your mind's ear to that first sound of new life.

Create a vivid visualisation of the exhilaration you feel as you see your baby at the moment of birth. See the three of you bonding for the first time in this life. Now mentally see yourself stepping into this joyful scene. Become a part of this birthing . . . fulfilled. Feel it . . . sense it. This is your body, here, now. In your mind's eye, see and feel yourself totally enveloping that body . . . holding the baby on your breast. These are your arms enfolding your baby; these are your hands embracing this new little being.

You knew you could do it, and you did. You did well, and the feeling of ecstasy is one that will never be surpassed.

Join in with joy and amazement and watch the continuing mystery of creation unfold. The life force of nature is working in harmony with you. Now more than at any moment in your life, it is within you and with you. You are an integral part of nature, and nature is an integral part of your being. You are a part of the greatest celebration of life. You are a part of the promise and the destiny of life itself.

The Opening Blossom

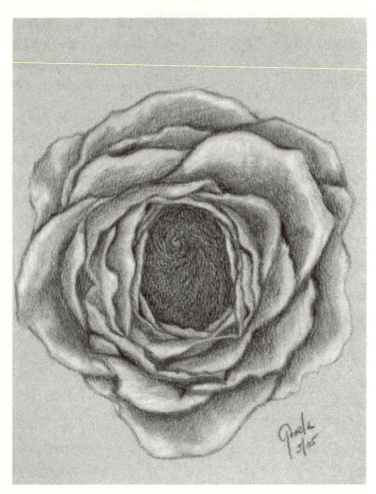

One of the most simple and effective visualisations is that of an opening rose. Use your breathing techniques to bring yourself into relaxation, then close your eyes and envision your baby moving gently down to the vaginal outlet. Imagine the gradual opening of the perineum to be like the gentle unfolding of the petals of the rose. This visualisation is recommended during the final days of your pregnancy to achieve the onset of labour, and also during the opening and birthing phases of labour.

Blue Satin Ribbons

Remember the lower circular muscle fibres that are drawn up and back to effect the thinning and opening of your cervix? Close your eyes and imagine the muscles not as fibres, but as soft, blue satin ribbons that gently and easily yield to the rhythmic draw of the vertical muscles, swirling up and back. You can practise this visualisation toward the end of your pregnancy so that it will be there for you during the surges of the thinning and opening phase of your labour.

The Arm-Wrist Relaxation Test

Because you don't really experience a particular sensation when you are in self-hypnosis, you will be amused and amazed at the Arm-Wrist Relaxation Test. It is very simple and, at the same time, very convincing. The technique is meant to assure both the birth companion and the mum that all the practice that you've been doing is working.

The Arm-Wrist Relaxation Technique

Lie on your back, with your arms at your side, your fingers gently cupped on the surface of the bed or sofa. Do not lie flat on your back for long periods of time or when you are in the late stages of pregnancy or in labour.

Once you are in a state of relaxation, picture that your birth companion has tied a giant, helium-filled red balloon to your right wrist. Almost immediately you will feel a tug on your wrist as the balloon

pulls upward. Now another helium-filled balloon—this one orange—
is added. The two balloons are tugging even harder on your wrist.
Your arm is beginning to rise upward. You sense that your elbow is
making a dent in the cushion or surface of your bed. The deeper the
dent, the more your wrist moves upward. With each tug, your arm is
being pulled higher. Still another balloon—a yellow one—is being
added. Each time a balloon is added, your arm begins to feel lighter
and lighter. The more you try to hold your wrist down, the more the
helium is pulling your arm upward. Your arm cannot resist the pull
of the balloons. Try as you may to hold it down, your wrist is being
yanked upward. Continue to picture more balloons being added with
all of the colours of the rainbow.

When your arm rises approximately six to ten inches off the bed,
place it back at your side. Each time you practise this exercise, fewer
balloons will be required to make your arm and wrist tilt upward.
At the end of each relaxation period, tell yourself that each time you
practise, relaxation will take over your body sooner than ever before.
Your goal should be to assume a deep level of relaxation within a very
short period of time.

Ultra-Deepening Techniques

These techniques have been found to be extremely effective in deepening relaxation to a point where the mother's body is totally limp, and she is in an almost amnesiac state. The expanded sessions of these exercises that you will practise in class with your practitioner will help you achieve the deep level of relaxation that you will use when you are nearing completion and beginning to use gentle Birth Breathing. This total relaxation allows the mum to go within to her birthing body and her baby. Often a mother will remain in this deep state while she breathes her baby down the birth path to the time for the baby to emerge.

To practise this combination of techniques, just breathe yourself into a state of relaxation. Once your body feels comfortably limp, you are ready to proceed.

Glove Relaxation

Glove Relaxation is the first of a combination of deepening techniques, and it is one of the best ways for you and your birth companion to plant an anchor for deep, soothing relaxation. It is also quite effective as a directive during labour and birthing. For this reason, I recommend that it be one of the primary elements of your practice sessions.

Glove Relaxation Technique

Imagine that you are putting a soft, silver glove onto your right hand—a special glove of natural endorphins. Immediately the fingers of your hand begin to feel larger and to tingle, as though there were springs at the ends of your fingers. The silver glove, with its endorphins flowing around your fingers, your palm, and the back of your hand, will cause your hand to feel numb, the way it would if you were to place it into a large container of icy slush.

As your birth companion strokes the back of your hand and arm, feel a tingling and then a numbness surrounding your hand and moving up your arm. Once your hand and arm lose all sensation, they begin to seem as lifeless and senseless as a piece of wood or a piece of leather. The silver mist of endorphins gradually drifts throughout your hand so that it can be transferred wherever you wish to bring about relaxation and comfort. To transfer the numbing effect, just visualise placing your hand on various parts of your body—each part now feels light, numb, and senseless. Even mothers who claim to feel uncomfortable when being touched fall into relaxation when the birth companion uses this technique and recites birthing prompts.

Practice will condition your body to react with calm when you feel your hand and arm being stroked. Go only with your breathing and your visualisations, not your body. Let your body continue to lie totally limp and senseless.

The Depthomet

The purpose of this exercise is to have

yourself into an ultradeep state of relaxatic

during the latter part of the opening phase o

and now

as th

The Depthometer Technique

In your mind's eye, see or imagine within your body a large, soft, flexible, inverted thermometer. The bulb of the thermometer is just above your forehead. The flexible tube extends all the way down to your toes. Inside the bulb is a clear fluid of natural relaxation.

There are forty gradations on the thermometer. As you count down from 40 to 39 to 38, and so on, picture the fluid of relaxation gently flowing down from one number to the next, flowing out into your circulatory system and bringing your body into relaxation. To reinforce the concept of relaxation filling every cell, nerve, and muscle of your body, visualise more fluid flowing down into the tube of the thermometer. You will feel a deep relaxation gradually saturating your body as the fluid fills the space in the tube.

As you reach each descending decade number on the thermometer —30, 20, 10, and 0—you will experience the feeling of doubling your current relaxation as you go deeper. By the time you reach the lower teens, you will find yourself in a very deep relaxation. The final ten digits will bring you to the ultra-deep relaxation you will use during the latter part of the thinning and opening phase of labour.

When you reach this new ultradeep level you will find yourself in the control centre of your inner mind.

When your body is thoroughly relaxed, the feeling of calm flowing from the silver glove will drift around your wrist, your lower arm,

ll the way to your elbow. Your arm begins to feel almost
ugh it were not there. Once you experience this sensation, the
laxation can be transferred to other parts of your body, particularly
the lower pelvic area. You can use this visualisation alone or with your
birthing companion in practice or during labour.

The Sensory Gate Control Valve

While still in your inner control room, look around you, and you'll
see in your mind's eye a large control panel with many lights and
switches. In the middle of that panel is a large round valve, and above
the valve are the words "HypnoBirthing Valve."

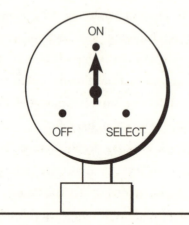

The Sensory Gate Control Valve

The Sensory Gate Valve Technique

This valve controls the messages that are sent from the brain past the
sensory gate in the brain stem to all of the nerves in your body. You
can use the indicator switch on this valve to shut off feeling throughout

your body. Simply see yourself turning the switch on the valve to the "off" position at eight o'clock.

This imagery, combined with the Glove relaxation, helps to bring about a loss of sensation in selected parts of your body. The imagery of the control valve can be used for any number of things, such as keeping your blood pressure at a safe and healthy level, maintaining a safe amount of amniotic fluid and controlling your stress level. You might want to give it a test by suggesting to yourself that your right foot is just too numb and heavy. No matter how hard you try, it does not want to lift; it is stuck to the floor.

Be sure to return the switch to the off position and release all self-hypnosis and restore all normal functions to your body before attempting to move about.

You will experience practise with an additional ultra-depth for birthing script in your HypnoBirthing class session.

Time Distortion

We know that people who experience hypnosis rarely have a good sense of the length of time that they are in a session. This is a blessing to the birthing mother.

Once you have mastered the art of bringing yourself into relaxation, you may want to begin practising time distortion. When you are in a relaxed state, give yourself the suggestion that every five minutes will seem as one minute. During labour, when you are nearing the end of your thinning and opening phase, the birth companion will give you the suggestion that every twenty minutes will seem as five. Time distortion is an important part of birthing and is included among the prompts used by the birth companion.

This loss of a sense of time, and the accompanying state of amnesia, comes at a time in labour when you are so deeply relaxed that it is difficult for you to talk, and you lose a sense of the people around you. At this time, you will go more deeply into your birthing body and to your baby, and you will begin your journey together. This is a gift of nature that can occur with all birthings if the mother is willing to let go, bring herself deep enough, and turn her birthing over to her birthing instinct and her baby.

---

*The partner's encouragement and
practical help increase the effectiveness of
labour-coping techniques, such as creative imagery and
breathing patterns. The presence also increases the
woman's chance of an emotionally fulfilling birth.*

Carl Jones, *The Birth Partner's Handbook*

Nutrition

Contributions by Dr. Charles Swencionis

W e've talked about the emotional, mental, and psychological aspects of birthing. These are all important to help you achieve a calm and relaxed birthing. But what you put into your body in the way of nutrition and how you prepare your body physically for birthing can make all the difference in the world in how your birthing plays out. Good nutrition is essential if you hope to have a healthy pregnancy and healthy birth and intend to sidestep many of the special circumstances of late pregnancy that can turn your birthing around.

Water: The Miracle Liquid

Consuming a sufficient amount of water is one of the most important elements in your daily health routine during pregnancy, and it's one of the easiest tasks that you can fit into your schedule. You need to consume water and other liquids, such as juices, to keep your body hydrated for better all-around bodily function. Hydration is paramount.

Approximately 60 percent of the human body is composed of water. It is one of the chief means of transportation within the body, carrying essential nutrients to the tissues and muscles that need them. Water aids in your digestion by moving food through the digestive system and then moving toxic waste products out of your body in elimination—two very important considerations when you are pregnant. Water acts as a lubricant, as well as a cushion for joints and muscles, and plays a major role in the spinal cord. It also helps to maintain a healthy body temperature. Because pregnancy changes the way your body stores and uses fluids, the kidneys are far more active in filtering toxins. Increasing your consumption of water can aid in this process and help avoid problems with toxemia later in pregnancy.

Water is one of the least expensive ways to maintain good physical health during your pregnancy, and it will help to ensure that you don't experience some of the inconveniences that some pregnant women may encounter, such as joint pain, constipation, muscle cramps, digestive problems, and a host of other common annoyances. It is far better to avoid these nuisances than to require steps to treat them.

Water is continually lost through exertion and body heat, as well as through the skin, kidneys, lungs, colon, and urination and perspiration. When you lose water through these means, it needs to be replaced because of the body's need for water. Amniotic fluid is replenished at least three times a day.

You will read and hear many recommendations concerning the amount of water that a pregnant woman should consume. Generally, it is recommended that a pregnant woman drink eight medium (200ml)glasses of water daily. You will need to consume more water if your activity level is high; if you live in a higher elevation; if the air where you live is less humid; if air temperatures are high; or if you consume a high-fibre diet; which you may be doing to ward off constipation.

The current thinking in determining how much water you should drink is simple. Allow your body to tell you what it needs, as it so nicely does in many other circumstances. You can easily tell if you are consuming a sufficient amount of water by checking the colour of your urine. A body that is properly hydrated releases urine that is the colour of light lemonade. If your urine is a deeper yellow, you need to reach for water more regularly and increase your consumption of protein. Pregnancy vitamins can affect the colour of your urine, so you will want to take that into consideration when assessing your colour. It's that simple.

You will also want to be aware of the quality of water—clean spring water or filtered water is optimal. Being faithful to this regimen can help prevent numerous pregnancy problems, as well as dry skin and other complexion problems.

Eating for Two

No single issue is more important as you carry your baby than the nutrition you provide for him as he develops and grows. You are building another little person made of bones, organs, tissues, muscles, blood, and cells. It doesn't matter how conscientiously you approach any building task and how carefully you think you're building, if the materials that go into the construction are less than the best, your project could prove to be less successful than you would like to see. Building a human being is even more exacting. There needs to be more attention paid to nutrition during the birthing year, and next to nothing is focused on nutrition prior to conception, so now is the time to take responsibility for good nutrition for your baby.

Since the HypnoBirthing philosophy is also one of avoiding late-term consequences of a poor diet, we have set down a few general suggestions that will help you and your baby to maintain good health. It takes a healthy mother to have a healthy baby. Healthy mothers have fewer low-birthweight infants, fewer incidences of premature birth, fewer cases of PIH (pregnancy-induced hypertension) or simply high blood pressure, and fewer incidences of toxemia. (The last two are generally lumped together, though not accurately, and known as preeclampsia.) In general, the pregnancies and births of healthy mothers are more apt to be "normal." The way to start on the road to good pregnancy health, no matter where you are in your pregnancy, is to realise that you are the single source of nutrition for your baby. If he is going to be well nourished, it's going to have to be through you.

Of course, pregnancy vitamin supplements are fine, but they are just that—supplements—which means that you should consume them in addition to a wholly nutritious diet, not as a substitute for a good food programme. It also means that, like most of the population, when you do your grocery shopping, you have to do it defensively. Buy fresh and organic foods as often as possible, rather than processed foods, and become educated as to which fruits and vegetables may have been sprayed with pesticides or treated with preservatives. As with everything in your pregnancy, ask questions. You need to protect your baby.

Note: Though these suggestions have been reviewed by a dietician and have been suggested by nutritionists, if you are experiencing a pregnancy that has special circumstances attached or if you have special food considerations, you will want to consult a nutritionist or dietician rather than follow the course of our suggestions. With no intent to offend those who follow a vegetarian and vegan diet, I will leave those matters to the people who subscribe to that diet and who are far more knowledgeable than I in this matter.

Basic Formula for Good Nutrition

- Drink water

- Eat veggies!

- Eat at least 75–100 grams of protein a day.

- Be sure the fats you eat are mostly natural. Avoid processed industrial oils such as vegetable oil.

- Eat whole foods. Avoid processed foods that come in boxes and bags, and "wipe out whites": Eat no white food unless it's protein. This includes breads, rice, sugar, flour, white baked goods, and starches.

A Note on Food Quality

Let's focus on the nourishing foods we should eat. And while it's important to eat the right food groups, it's also essential to pay attention to food quality. Under each of the five main points below, we've included notes for selecting quality foods that will best nourish your baby while you are pregnant.

Pursuing perfection can be stressful, and therefore counterproductive for a healthy pregnancy. So do the best you can. Even if you incorporate one or two things from this chapter into your diet, you will be doing a service to your baby and yourself.

If you are interested in looking further, here are some resources for exploring this topic:

Deep Nutrition by Catherine Sahanahan, M.D.
Real Food and Real Food for Mum and Baby by Nina Planck
The Better Baby Book by Dave and Lana Asprey
Beautiful Babies by Kristen Michaelis
Food Rules, The Omnivore's Dilemma, and *Cooked* by Michael Pollan
It Starts With Food by Dallas and Melissa Hartwig
Nourishing Traditions by Sally Fallon and Mary Enig

Organic produce is preferable to conventionally farmed food if it is available and affordable. If not, keep in mind the "Clean 15" and the "Dirty Dozen."

The "Clean 15" foods have skins that chemicals can't penetrate easily; once washed and peeled, they can be safely eaten. These include: onions, avocados, sweet corn, pineapples, asparagus, cabbage, aubergine, grapefruit, sweet peas, kiwi, cantaloupe, watermelon, sweet potatoes, mango, and papayas.

The "Dirty Dozen" have skins that chemicals can penetrate easily; washing and peeling them won't necessarily remove the chemicals. These include: peaches; celery; strawberries; apples; spinach, kale and lettuce; potatoes, blueberries, nectarines, sweet bell peppers, cherries, cucumbers, and grapes.

High-quality proteins have proportions of amino acids that make building human tissue easy. Complete protein is possible by combining vegetables and grains. When we think of protein, we usually think of muscle meats and eggs, and that's true; those are excellent sources of high-quality, complete proteins.

But the ingredients for growing happy, healthy babies are found in a variety of healthy foods from each of the food groups. You should plan to increase your daily calorie intake by about 300 calories. Here are a few suggestions:

Eat:

Lots of protein—75 to 100 grams a day, taken in several snacks or light meals. Protein is the cornerstone of your nutrition programme. Protein includes such food items as cottage cheese, milk, ice cream, frozen yogurt, cheeses (except soft cheeses like Camembert, brie, and Roquefort), safe fish (see information to follow), peanut butter, lean red meat, poultry, pork, ham, bacon, lamb, veal tofu, eggs, butter, rabbit, vegetables, nuts and seeds (high sources), and fruits.

Celtic, Mediterranean, Pink Himalayan sea salt—with no minerals removed (salt your food to taste).

Safe fish—Increase your intake of safe fish or fish oils, which contain omega-3. Check before buying for possible mercury risks. (Don't eat raw fish.)

Green foods—dark, leafy raw foods, celery, green peppers, apples, broccoli, peas, avocado, string beans, Brussels sprouts, asparagus, broccoli, lima beans, collard greens, Swiss chard, grapes, limes, beet greens, courgettes, dandelion greens, lettuce, spinach (only occasionally as it can limit the absorption of calcium), watercress, snow peas.

It is believed that the darker and brighter the fruits and vegetables, the more nutrition they deliver.

Vegetables—Evidence suggests that children whose mothers ate more vegetables while pregnant found vegetables more palatable and had fewer aversions to eating vegetables later in childhood, setting up healthy habits for the years to come.

Orange foods—squash, yams and sweet potatoes, cantaloupe, oranges, peaches, apricots, nectarines, pumpkin, tangerines, carrots, peppers (raw and cooked).

Red foods—watermelon, strawberries (if not sprayed with pesticides), peppers (raw or cooked), tomatoes, apples, raspberries (drink red raspberry leaf tea), cherries, rhubarb, red potatoes, pimiento, radishes.

Coloured fruits—pineapple, pears, bananas, honeydew melons, kiwi, grapes.

Avoid:

- **Alcohol**

- **Caffeine**

- **Nicotine**

- **Processed meats**—hot dogs, luncheon meats, bologna, liverwurst.

- **Raw fish**—oysters, sushi, and others.

- **Unnecessary fats**—fried foods, French fries, fast foods.

- **White foods**—refined sugar, white flour products, white rice, white potatoes.

- **Sweets**—candies with empty calories that have no nutritional value.

Exercising and Toning

It is particularly important that you exercise during pregnancy. It is also crucial, however, that you don't build exercising into a routine that becomes an ordeal or a time-consuming chore. You will want to find ways to tone your body that are as natural as the birthing you are preparing for. Vary the exercises that you do and create a habit of doing them as often as you can as you go about your day-to-day activities.

You'll discover that many exercises can be practised incidentally. Some can even be done right on your bed as you awaken in the morning or just before you settle in for the night. If you are accustomed to brisk exercise, consult with your care provider to be sure that this kind of exercise will not compromise your baby's well-being.

One of the best ways to ensure that you are exercising regularly is to join a prenatal fitness and exercise group. Most of the time, the mothers in these classes are pretty upbeat about their pregnancies and upcoming birthings. Avoid any group that is given to commiserating over bad birth stories.

HypnoBirthing

188   *HypnoBirthing*

Walking

Walking is one of the best exercises you can do. It helps to strengthen your breathing, as well as your legs. You don't have to follow a strict regimen of walking, but you can look for ways to get in a little extra walking time, for example, by parking a distance from the entrance to your work or from the supermarket. Use an entrance that is not immediately adjacent to your destination. Rather than telephoning or taking an elevator to another area, find occasions to walk within the building at work. Walk as often as you can. Be sure that the surfaces you walk on are smooth and safe, and wear sensible shoes. Brisk walking is good from the beginning to the middle of your pregnancy. After that you may want to slow down a bit so that your baby is not jostled too much. When you engage in brisk exercise, your blood is directed to your arms and legs and away from the uterus, meaning that your baby is perhaps not receiving the amount of oxygenated blood that he should. Temper your time and pace.

Avoid Back Strain: Practise Good Posture

As your pregnancy advances, you will want to alleviate back strain by being aware of correct posture. Pregnant or not, a good assist to proper posture is to envision a string passing from a point at the front of the earlobe down through the shoulders and the hipbone to a spot just behind the ankle bone. Keeping your head in line with this imaginary string will prevent you from "leading with your head," and keep your pelvis tilted back and help you to avoid stooping as you gain in weight and size.

Don't lean back with your head behind the imaginary line; it will cause you to project your abdomen forward and will lead to the "pregnancy waddle." Many women assume this posture, with toes turned outward, as depicted in comedy skits and sitcoms, long before final "dropping" has occurred. Even then, awareness of how you carry yourself and your baby can make a difference in how you feel at the end of a day.

One of the best devices for maintaining good posture and for helping to ensure that your baby will assume a favourable position for birthing is to avoid slouching down into your pelvic area. This is not too easy to do with so many cars being equipped with bucket seats today, but it can be remedied by placing a pillow on the seat so that it is more level. Absolutely avoiding recliners is also good advice for the pregnant woman who is interested in achieving an optimal position for her baby at birth.

One of the best ways to practise good posture when sitting is to regularly sit on a birth ball (also known as an exercise ball). These handy balls can be bought at any number of locations, including most sporting goods stores, at very reasonable prices. The birth ball allows you to sit erect and, at the same time, tones your inner thighs and pelvic region. Use it at your desk or as a place to relax at home, instead of a chair. The birth ball comes in handy later in pregnancy, and it is a great place to rock during labour. It is one of the best and simplest tools you can buy. To ensure good balance while using the birth ball, fill the bottom of the ball with approximately 2 inches of sand. This will prevent your tilting one way or another and help you maintain that erect posture that is so important.

Another exercise that is helpful in relieving back strain is the "pelvic rock." This exercise helps to avoid back strain, strengthens abdominal muscles, increases the flexibility of your lower back, and promotes good alignment in your spine. There are several ways to do the pelvic rock. Instructions for two methods follow.

First Method: Using the back of a sturdy chair or other piece of furniture for arm support and balance, stand approximately two feet from the object. Bend your knees very slightly.

Lean forward from your hips and thrust your buttocks backward. Keep your back straight. Allow your abdominal muscles to relax for a few seconds while you create sway.

Bend your knees a little more and pull your hips forward, tucking your buttocks under as though you were being shooed from behind with a broom. Repeat the procedure several times.

Second Method: You can also practise the pelvic rock or tilt in a lying position during the early months of your pregnancy. Once your baby begins to take on some weight, you will want to avoid lying flat on your back.

On your back with your knees bent and your feet flat on the floor, tighten your lower abdominal muscles and the muscles of your buttocks. Your tailbone will rise, pressing the small of your back to the floor. Hold this position for a few seconds and then release the muscles. As you do this exercise, arch your back as much as you can. Repeat the procedure several times.

You will also find this an excellent technique for flattening the abdomen following birthing.

Toning the Inner Thigh and Leg Muscles

Toning your inner thigh muscles and legs is vitally important for a successful labour. At the end of your birthing when you are breathing your baby down and out of the birth path, you may find yourself in many positions that will call for you to use your legs in ways that are a bit unusual. The muscles in your inner thigh will need to be ready.

Position One: The best effect in toning can be derived from sitting on the floor or in the middle of a bed with soles of your feet together. Lean slightly forward and place your hands on your ankles. With your elbows resting on the inside of your knees, gently press your elbows onto your knees. Do not apply force as you stretch these important groin muscles. As you do these exercises over time, gradually and gently pull your heels toward your crotch until your heels and your crotch meet and your knees almost rest on the floor. Do not rush to make this happen. Take it slowly. Once you have achieved this muscle tone, you should straighten your back during subsequent practise sessions.

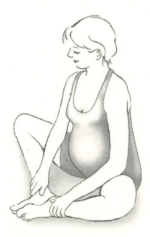

Toning the Inner Thigh Muscles

You can do this exercise alone, but it's more fun to get your birthing companion involved. Using the same technique as described previously, have the birth companion assist from behind you by placing his or her hands under your knees, pressing upward to create resistance. While this is happening, you gently press down on your knees. Then have your birth companion press downward on your knees while you bring your legs upward and push against the pressure.

Position Two: Resting on your tailbone with your knees bent and raised upward toward your shoulders, place the palms of your hands against the inner part of your knees and push your knees outward. Bring your knees together again and then push them apart. Do this about ten times in each practice session.

When you reach for low objects or lift an object or a small child, bend with your knees, rather than from the waist. Do not attempt to lift heavy objects.

The Leaping Frog

The Leaping Frog position comes to us from midwives in the Virgin Islands. This easy, forward squat is used in many places in the world. Not only does this position help to tone your muscles, but it also provides you with one of the best positions in which to labour during the birthing phase.

While women in other cultures regularly use a squatting position for birthing, you must remember that these women use this posture for much of what they do on a daily basis. Western women are not naturally inclined to squatting, so this posture needs practice. There are two ways of assuming the Leaping Frog stance—with your arms thrust forward inside your spread knees or with your arms behind you at the side of your hips. The second position is an ideal position to assume for birthing as it relieves all pressure from the buttocks and provides open and clear access for both baby and attendant. The time that you spend in practising this modified form of squatting will be well spent.

Assuming the Leaping Frog position during labour offers benefits for both you and your baby when you are Birth Breathing. Just a few of the benefits of the Leaping Frog include the following:

- Widens the pelvic opening

- Relaxes and opens the perineal tissues

- Helps to avoid tearing and lessens the need for an episiotomy

- Relieves strain in the lower back

- Increases the supply of oxygen to your baby

- Shortens the birth path

- Allows you a clear view of your baby's birth

- Makes good use of the effect of gravity

Though I recommend the Leaping Frog position, attempting to adopt it for any length of time when your muscles are not adequately toned could result in pain or injury to your leg muscles. If you choose to birth with your arms behind you, you will want considerable practice so that your arms will be able to support you. A variation of this is to lean with your arms on your companion's knees so that you can slowly lower yourself into the squatting position. The companion can also stand in front of you, holding your hands to assist as you slowly lower your body into position.

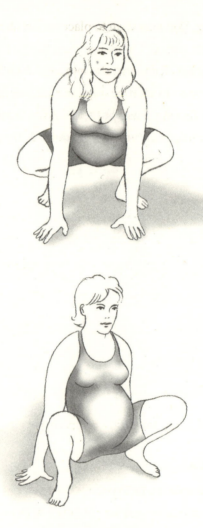

Leaping Frog Positions

From a standing position with your feet spread about a foot and a half apart, assume a squatting position on your toes with your knees spread outward. Place your hands on the floor on either the inside or the outside of your legs.

During birthing, you may wish to place pillows beneath your hands and your knees.

This same position nicely converts into a Polar Bear position if there is need to assist baby to shift position during birthing. This is easily accomplished by leaning your chin and your forearms on the pillows in front of you, while your buttocks extend into the air.

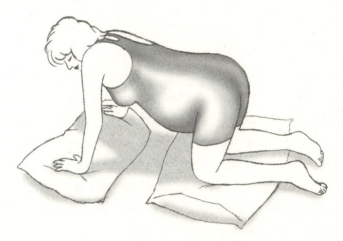

Hands and knees position

Pelvic Floor Exercises

Not enough attention is paid to pelvic floor exercises, sometimes called Kegels. They are among the most important of all the prenatal muscle toning. Designed to tone and strengthen the muscles used during the birthing phase of labour, these exercises involve the network of muscles that form a figure eight around the entire vaginal and anal region.

Toning the pelvic floor muscles also serves the very important function of quick return to their normal size after labour and can be helpful in preventing some of the urinary problems connected with aging.

Control of this area can actually enhance lovemaking after having a child. You will enjoy the confidence derived from a well-toned anal and vaginal region as your pregnancy advances and there is more pressure on the bladder and bowel. These sphincters are the same sphincters that you will use while practising Birth Breathing on the toilet. As you breathe down, you will want to open both the vaginal and anal outlets, keeping them open during the intake of the next soft breath.

Technique

In a sitting position, start by constricting the lowest muscles of the anal and vaginal tracts as tightly as you can. Keep tightening the vaginal muscles until you can feel the constricting muscles all the way up into the top of the vagina. When working with anal muscles, draw in until you get the sensation of pulling the anus into the rectum. It is helpful, though not necessary, to count from one to ten as you do these exercises, tightening a little more with each number. When you have tightened the muscles in the area, hold the contraction for a few seconds and then release slowly.

These muscles are the same ones used to stop the flow of urine. To see if you are doing this exercise correctly, attempt to stop the flow of urine while you are urinating. Do not continue to do this once you have established that you are doing the exercise correctly. To do this more than is necessary could result in a urinary tract infection. Be sure to practise this exercise several times a day, doing the exercise five to ten times at each practise. Frequent practice is all to your benefit. These exercises can be done easily at anytime, anywhere, whether at work or at home, while driving or while walking. The important thing is to DO IT.

Perineal Massage

erineal massage is one of the oldest and surest ways of improving the health, blood flow, elasticity, and relaxation of the pelvic floor muscles. Practised in the latter part of your pregnancy, approximately six to eight weeks prior to term, this technique will also help you to identify and become acquainted with the tissues you will relax and the region through which you will birth your baby. Perineal massage is vitally important to the success of your HypnoBirthing. Do not take this exercise for granted.

Massaging with oil helps the perineal tissues to soften and thereby gently unfold with no resistance as they open during birthing to allow the passage of the baby. As you or your partner do the massage, you can teach these muscles to relax and open outward in response to pressure.

This massage increases your chances of birthing your baby over an intact perineum. When your perineal rim is soft and relaxed, the perennial folds easily open, and your baby slips past the rim and out of the vagina. The perenial tissues gently unfold. Attention to this massage will pay off. It is simple, yet so effective. You will want to take it seriously. The massage should be done every day for at least five minutes.

Because of your increased size and the awkwardness of bending around your abdomen, it may be easier to have someone else do the massage for you. If the massage is done gently, there is no need for discomfort. I suggest that couples make it part of their lovemaking.

If you are doing the massage by yourself, you'll find it easier if you use your thumb. Place one foot on the seat of a chair, with the other approximately two feet away from the chair. This allows you to work around and under your abdomen from the back.

Be sure that fingernails are smooth and short when doing the massage. A rubber glove will ensure that there are no rough surfaces to irritate the vaginal tissue. You may use virgin olive oil, sweet oil, almond oil, apricot oil, or a lubricating gel. Avoid perfumed oils.

Technique

Pour a little of the oil into a custard cup or shallow bowl. (Be sure to discard oil that is left after massaging—do not reuse.)

Sit with your back resting against pillows and get comfortable. It's a good idea to use a mirror during the first few times that you do this exercise. It will assist you in identifying the muscles involved and allow you to observe the easing of the edge of the perineum.

Dip your thumb into the oil and thoroughly moisten it. If a partner is doing the massage, the first two fingers will be used. The thumb or fingers should be dipped into the oil to the second knuckle and inserted into the vagina approximately two to three inches, pressing downward on the area between the vagina and the rectum. Rub the oil into the inner edge of the perineum and the lower vaginal wall.

Maintaining a steady pressure, slide the fingers upward along the sides of the vagina in a U, sling-type motion. This pressure will stretch the vaginal tissue, the muscles surrounding the vagina, and the outer rim of the perineum. Be sure to reach the inner portions as well as the outer rim of the perineum. In the beginning you will feel the tightness of the muscles, but with time and practice, the tissue will relax.

Practise relaxing the extended muscles by picturing the perineum opening outward as pressure is applied. The opening rosebud is a good visualisation to use during this exercise.

Selecting Your Care Providers

Birth is the last frontier in a woman's
quest for freedom. A woman needs to be free to
birth her babies as she chooses.

Lorne Campbell, Sr., M.D.

You Can't Grow Orchids in the Arctic

You probably have never given much thought to growing orchids; but for the sake of conversation, let's assume that you have decided to devote your life to growing orchids. Without any in-depth thought as to the people you will work with or the surroundings in which you will be working, you choose to take your project to the Arctic Circle.

It will not be long after your plane touches down that you discover that the Arctic is little more than large, barren fields of ice. The people who brought you there confirm that the Arctic is no place to grow orchids. The freezing temperatures offer a bitter cold welcome. You know that you've made a huge mistake. The Arctic is definitely not conducive to your fulfilling of your dream to grow orchids. So you leave, saddened and disappointed but not defeated.

When you get home, a little bit of inquiry and research clearly indicates that Singapore would have been the better choice. The people there are entirely supportive, and the surroundings and environment are conducive to growing orchids. So you confidently take your seedlings and head for Singapore convinced that Singapore is all you are looking for.

Approaching your upcoming birthing day without exploring these same factors—the attitudes of the people who will attend you, the physical surroundings and the general environment of your birth facility—is not unlike attempting to grow orchids in the Arctic.

This is your baby's first birthday, and as a parent, it is your responsibility to do all you can to ensure that the right people attend the birth and that the birthing facility is a perfect match for the birth you are envisioning. All other decisions that you will be making will pale in comparison to the importance of these factors. The most important question you must ask yourself is "How certain am I that my primary birth attendant will listen to my requests and honour me and my baby as a birthing family?" The philosophy and management style of this person and the policies and procedures in effect at the facility are the most essential.

Parents often will ask "But how can I find that really caring birth professional?" We say listen and pay attention to your gut sense. If it feels right, you have found the right person. If when you leave the provider's office, you feel anything less than enthusiastic about this person, your inner knowing is sending you a message.

A member of the HypnoBirthing faculty, Lori Nicholson, of Bethesda, Maryland, offers the following thought-provoking scenario to her parent classes. She suggests this approach:

Imagine yourself employed in an important position in a fairly large organisation. The Chief Administrative Officer of the organisation has called you into his office to explain that he is interested in becoming involved in an important project that will require hiring a key person to oversee this project. He is appointing you to act as the hiring manager.

The first candidate whom you interview starts the interview by telling you that he is very familiar with the project but feels that its objectives are flawed. He feels that the project has very little likelihood of success and suggests that his approach should be adopted. He states that he is very well educated, and he has good experience and a good work history. He has a good personality and feels that he is the person for this job of Project Overseer. Based on your conversation with this person, would you hire him for this job? Would he be the person that you feel you could trust to bring about a successful and happy conclusion?

As a parent of your unborn baby, you are the hiring manager whose job it is to select the very best person for the position of the overseer of your birthing. The person you select can either make or break the success of the birthing day.

As birthing parents, you can achieve that freedom only when you take responsibility for seeing that the people you surround yourselves with are people who hold the same view of birth as you do and who are willing to respect and support your dreams. You do have choices, and you need to identify them.

Even in an ideal situation, you may need to keep reminding the care-giver that you are planning for a HypnoBirthing. Mention your birth preferences early and often, without being irksome. Health-care providers are busy people who see many families. They sometimes need that gentle reminder.

If you've had a surgical birth previously and truly want to birth vaginally this time, seriously look into having a VBAC (vaginal birth after caesarean) and actively seek a doctor or midwife who will encourage you. The HypnoBirthing method is especially favourable to VBACs because the breathing techniques are gentle all through the opening phase, and you will not strain with forced pushing during the baby's descent—another plus for the VBAC mother.

Many providers who have never seen HypnoBirthing are more than happy to keep an open mind and support your wishes if the benefits are presented to them in an inviting, rather than demanding, way.

YOUR OPTIONS - AND YOU DO HAVE CHOICES

There is no one system of care that covers the entire UK. Several systems are in place; but it is true to say that midwife-led care is the norm for most healthy, low-risk women in the National Health Service (NHS). Midwives are considered the guardians of normal birth and will do their utmost to see that normal birth is achieved. Their philosophy is sometimes shared with the general practitioner; but, for the most part, it is the midwife who is seen as the birthing expert.

The clientele of the midwife is mostly healthy women in a low-risk category. However, midwives are trained to detect possible abnormalities and make an appropriate referral to a doctor.

There are choices for midwifery services. When making your decision, look into your heart, consider your birthing wishes, and be sure that you feel comfortable with your choice. The following options are legitimate from both a safety and comfort perspective:

Community Midwives: Community midwives are organised into groups of six to eight midwives. Their services include antenatal appointments at clinics in the community, as well as home visits for anywhere from 10 to 29 days following the birth of the baby. Women working with community midwives may choose to give birth at home, and will have an opportunity, in most cases, to meet the group of midwives prior to their birthings.

A small percentage of women who choose to birth in the local hospital will be cared for by a team member, the others will be cared for by a staff midwife at the hospital.

The idea of team midwifery is popular with women preparing to give birth since they are able to get to know the person who will attend their birth and they are able to discuss their preferences beforehand. Midwives are guided by the women's choices for birthing and are equally comfortable giving support to a woman wishing a fully natural birth, as with a woman who feels that she may need some degree of medication.

Midwife-led Birth Centres: Another option in some areas is an NHS midwife-led birth centre. These units are made as homelike as possible. They have pools for labour and/or birthing and are staffed solely by midwives and health-care assistants or maternity-care assistants.

Independent Midwives: The concept of working with an independent midwife is also another option. Independent midwives are trained by the NHS and must practice by their standards. Most support natural birth and encourage the use of a birthing pool and homeopathy to enhance the experience.

You may hire an independent midwife by contacting the midwife and arranging a private agreement for her services. The agreement may be dependent upon whether all or only part of the care is to be covered by the midwife, and fees are charged accordingly. (For more information visit www.imuk.org.uk.)

If your pregnancy is categorised as high risk, you will probably need to have a caregiver who attends births in the hospital.

Midwives work in close conjunction with physicians in the event that a birthing does require a medical referral. Midwives usually are quite receptive to listening and supporting the wishes of birthing parents, but this, too, can differ with individuals.

> *My three recent trips to England to teach HypnoBirthing certification classes have allowed me to observe an entirely different approach to birth than what we experience in the United States. It is interesting to note the attitude toward midwifery and birthing in the United Kingdom and contrast it with ours in the United States. In the United Kingdom, midwives are the principal attendants at births and have a legal obligation to attend a birthing mother wherever she wishes to birth. In the early 1990s, the House of Commons in the UK officially mandated that the needs of birthing mothers be the central focus of maternal health-care providers and that maternity services be fashioned around them, not the other way around. Refreshing!*

In the United Kingdom and other countries that operate under a National Health System (NHS), your birthing attendant could be one of any number of midwives. A midwife in the United Kingdom works with the NHS, serving women with normal pregnancies and labour. In addition to doing all of the antenatal clinics and attending births, he/she will also cover the postnatal period up to twenty-eight days. While their clientele is mostly healthy women in a low-risk category, midwives are trained to detect possible abnormalities and make an appropriate referral to a doctor. Under this system, healthy women with healthy pregnancies can be attended by midwives, and most women never need to see a doctor. Almost three quarters of women birthing in the Netherlands are attended by midwives.

One of my mums had her first baby last Sunday at home. She completed the course with me only two weeks earlier ... She went into labour spontaneously and called the homebirth midwife to come and check her because she was "getting some strange sensations"! The midwife stayed for an hour and concluded that there was no way the mum was in active labour. The midwife could not tell when the mum was having surges and had to ask her to indicate them by squeezing her husband's hand so that the baby could be monitored.

Baby and mother were so calm that the midwife said that she would leave them for a few hours and to call if things progressed. The mum then said, "Before you go, can you just tell me — is it normal to want to push at this stage?" The midwife was compelled to do an exam and found that the mum was fully open and the head was visible!! A beautiful baby boy was breathed into the world twenty minutes later.

Later, as the midwife was leaving, she said to a very ecstatic, proud and alert mum, "Well, I have never seen anything like that before. You are obviously made to have babies." To which the mum replied: "Yes, I'm a woman!"

Vanessa, Wales, U.K.

In some areas, you may have the option of a midwifery system
called the Domino scheme, whereby community midwives are
attached to a hospital. The Domino scheme provides the same con-
tinuity of care as for a home birth, but provides the opportunity for
a woman to give birth in hospital, if she feels that is where she will
be most comfortable. This option can mean that all antenatal services will be conducted by midwives, with the possibility of seeing
a different midwife at each visit. If your labour is prolonged or spills
from one shift to another, you could have more than one midwife
attend your birthing.

---

*I was in my fortieth week of pregnancy and had looked for-
ward to a planned homebirth, but a late test result indicated
that it couldn't be. I needed to change plans fast for birthing
with a midwife and seek a physician. I felt this would not be
an easy task at this late date.*

*I called my family physician, Dr. Barrett, and made an
appointment to see him on Friday morning. The man earned
high honours in my book for being willing to take me on as a
patient at exactly forty weeks. I knew him to be a wonderful
doctor and a very compassionate man.*

*Friday afternoon, I began to have surges. This was nothing
new to me, as I had had surges off and on for many weeks,
but these were two to three minutes apart and felt different.
We got packed, got into the car and headed for the hospital.*

*We arrived a little after 3:30 and were admitted. Much to
my delight, the surges continued to get longer and stronger.*

→

Our doula, Missy, showed up soon after. Our nurse was puzzled that I could walk, talk and smile through surges, and seemed flustered to think that I was going to birth without an epidural. She said that unless the cervix is changing, it isn't real labour. I'm sure that she didn't believe that I was in true labour — too quiet and too relaxed. She called Dr. Barrett when I declined to answer the questions on the pain scale and told him that I had a very bossy doula who was telling me that I could refuse things. He supported my position.

When my membranes released at 6:40, I began to feel pressure. Missy recognised the signs and felt that this was going to be a really short labour. Reluctantly the nurse called Dr. Barrett. As soon as he came into the room, I released and began to nudge the baby down. Two surges later, our baby was born. I held him in my arms and cried with happiness for love of him and relief that he was here, alive and healthy.

Dr. Barrett spent the next two hours with us, as did Missy. He personally secured warm blankets for me, made sure I had food, gave me his pager number and did all the sweet things you would expect from a good friend. He was supportive of all the things I wanted. I gave birth without an IV or medication, ate throughout labour and had no anaesthesia.

This birth was different from what I had envisioned and hoped for a few weeks earlier, but it was the birth that our baby needed, and a beautiful birth at that.

Melanie, Salt Lake City

Obstetrician: Obstetricians are medical doctors who have graduated from an accredited school of medicine and have completed two to three years of advanced study in the field of gynaecology and obstetrics. They are highly trained surgeons and are proficient at detecting, diagnosing and treating gynaecological and obstetrical problems that require specialised procedures. They are skilled specialists who are called upon when special circumstances arise in birthing that require specific medical or surgical procedures. Because they are prepared and trained for surgical births, they would be most likely to see a large number of mothers who are in the category of high risk.

Obstetricians see pregnant women for examinations, testing and other antenatal care, as well as postnatal checkups. If a surgical birth is deemed necessary, an obstetrician will perform the caesarean section. Obstetricians do not need backup from another surgeon, except in rare or unusual circumstances.

I was concerned that I might not find a doctor who would understand our wanting to birth naturally, but Dr. Adams was wonderful. He had never heard of HypnoBirthing, but asked if he could take our book home with him to share with his wife who is preparing to become a doula. He was very accepting of our birth preferences.

My "Guess Date" was May 6, and on May 11, with my blood pressure rising, our doctor suggested induction. I was already at 4 centimetres open, and he knew that labour was near.

➡

We arrived at the hospital at 7:00 the following morning. Dr. Adams said that he would rupture the membranes rather than give me something stronger.

We spent the day walking when I wasn't being monitored. My husband said that I looked like I was drugged because I was so relaxed. When a surge came, I simply stopped walking and talking and closed my eyes. I visualised waves rolling in and out on a beach.

I was 6 centimetres opened at 6:00 P.M., but I wasn't told what stage I was in. I didn't want to know.

At 7:00 P.M., I felt I needed to be checked. I asked the nurse not to tell me how open I was because I didn't want to be disappointed or to ruin my frame of mind. She checked and said, "Well, I'll say this. I need to call the doctor and tell him to come quickly." Our baby was on his way down. When I crowned, I pushed two or three times, and my baby was born. I had an eight-pound baby boy at 8:36 P.M.

Throughout the whole birthing, I felt about one second of pain. I was scared by the sensation of tearing. I had two tiny tears that healed in a couple of days.

I did not need to practise time distortion because the whole day was a blur. I couldn't believe that twelve hours had passed. Our doctor and the nurses were truly amazed.

Our baby is easygoing, a good sleeper and nurses well, which I attribute to his calm, drug-free birth.

Thanks to a supportive doctor and to our HypnoBirthing practitioner for a miracle to be treasured always.

Teresa, Vermont

Here are a few questions you might ask the person(s) you are considering selecting to get a feel for their openness to normal birthing:

- We are planning to do HypnoBirthing — a natural birth; will you support us in that?

- How often do you perform caesarean births? What is the most common reason?

- Considering ten of your patients, how many do you feel will need to be induced? Need augmentation? Have a caesarean section?

- If our baby is strong, and I am fine, will you postpone discussion of induction until forty-two weeks?

- If release of membranes is the first sign of labour, how long are you willing to wait for spontaneous onset of labour? Why do you choose that number?

- During the birthing phase, I will be breathing the baby down to birth rather than forcefully pushing. Are you comfortable with that?

- I would like to eat light snacks for energy while in labour. What is your feeling about that?

Doula: A doula is a person who knows birthing and, from behind the scenes, helps parents achieve the uninterrupted birth they are seeking. A doula frees the birth companion to focus his or her attention upon the mum, while the doula tends to details of seeing that the mum has a cool facecloth that is refreshed regularly and reminds her to change positions or to empty her bladder. One of the most important roles that a doula plays is that of liaison with hospital staff when parents have a request or need help interpreting the situation. Just the presence of a doula helps to avoid the suggestion of intervention and allows parents to relax in the confidence that they are in good hands. (For more information on hiring a doula, visit www.doula.org.uk.)

Preparing Birth Preferences

Birth in a Sanctuary? Why not!

Imagine . . .
  A place where everyone
  Honours you and the work you will
    do in labour,
  Speaks quietly and moves slowly
    and gently,
  Respects your need to be spontaneous—
    to eat, drink, make sounds, move around, cry, shout, laugh,
  Treats you and your baby as fully conscious and sensitive beings.
  Giving birth is as intimate as lovemaking
    You will need privacy and support and tenderness
  Labour is not a spectator sport
    Your partner is not your "coach"
  It's the journey of a lifetime for your baby and you
    Don't settle for a typical birth
  Find out more . . . home birth . . . birth centres
    Safe alternatives to epidurals . . . Seek out a midwife
    Arrange for a labour companion/doula to stay with you . . .
Protect your baby and empower yourself!

SUZANNE ARMS

CHOOSING YOUR BIRTHING ENVIRONMENT

In-Hospital Birth Centres: Some hospitals have an entire unit devoted to birthing and the care of newborn babies — these are midwifery-led units. They have discarded the old "Labour and Delivery" signs and replaced them with names that indicate a softer, less medicalised atmosphere. A great deal of money and effort have been put into making these units appear attractive, comfortable and homelike. This is very appealing, but you must evaluate more than the decor. Matching curtains and bedspreads give an air of charm and a homelike appearance, but unless the people who come into this setting to attend the birthing families have a matching attitude of kindness, are family-oriented and view birth as normal, the decor becomes only window dressing, disguising the equipment, instruments and machinery that may be in full force during your birthing.

Supporting the belief that healthy women with healthy babies can safely birth outside the "geared-for-emergency" protocol, there are hospitals that are truly committed to natural birthing and family-friendly care and attention. Some of them have even allocated a sizeable segment of the birthing unit, and in some cases an entire floor, to families who want to birth naturally. These rooms are free of monitors and other medical equipment and apparatus. Mums are not immediately stripped of their clothing, put to bed, strapped to a machine and outfitted with an IV. Staff members are carefully selected to support the families who choose to birth there.

A hospital in Rochester, New Hampshire, is so commit-ted to gentle birth that nearly half of all of their births are HypnoBirthings. Thanks to the efforts of caring nurses and administrators, as well as the goodwill of a few HypnoBirth-ing practitioners, a hospital in San Diego, California, has an entire floor devoted to families who want to birth in an atmosphere that is as close to normal as possible. A large hos-pital in Chicago has an ABC unit (Alternative Birth Center), as do many others across the country. The trend is growing. You will want to be sure that the hospital you select is truly HypnoBirthing-friendly, lending an atmosphere that says birth is normal and not an emergency waiting to happen.

William and Martha Sears, authors of The Birth Book, suggest that "parent power" is the answer to making care providers and hos-pital administrators more sensitive to this need. When millions of expectant families call the hospital of their choice and ask for such accommodations, including a staff that supports normal birth, it will happen. Parents need to be aware, however, that, on occasion, the same hospital that teaches gentle birthing in their childbirth classes may meet the couple with "routine" procedures when they arrive at the hospital to birth their baby. Parents need to address this inconsist-ency, and it is a good idea to set the stage early. Ask the caregivers and the hospital staff, as well as parents who have birthed in that facility, if the facility is family-friendly and endorses the belief of normal birth.

If possible, tour more than one birthing facility and talk with the staff, just as you did when you selected your medical care provider. The answers to these questions will tell you about the hospital's philosophy. It's a good idea to do this early: You may want to change your plans based on your findings. Don't wait until just before your birthing time to inquire about these things.

Here are some questions for you to consider:

- Is there flexibility in policies and willingness to accommodate HypnoBirthing preferences in the absence of special circumstances?

- Are there midwives on staff who are partial to natural birth?

- Do they have a pool?

- Do they have birthing balls or can you bring one?

- Will you be fed if your labour lingers? Are snacks available?

- Are you free to walk outside or within the hospital?

- May you remain in your own clothes during labour?

- Is immediate, skin-to-skin bonding time allowed with the baby?

- Are doulas welcome?

- Is there a provision for the partner and baby to stay in the same room as the mum?

- Are statistics on inductions, augmentations, epidurals and caesarean births available?

Free-standing Birth Centres: The birth centre is more likely to afford you the opportunity to birth without intervention. You will want to ask the same questions of a birth centre staff member as you do of hospital staff. Because the birth centre focus is on healthy women with healthy pregnancies, they don't have to be equipped with all of the high-tech apparatus that is needed for women with pregnancy complications. Birthing in a birth centre, however, is as safe as hospital birthing.

Homebirth: There is much misunderstanding and misinformation about homebirths. Among them are the myths that homebirthing is dangerous while hospital births are safe.

A study done by Dr. Lewis Mehl-Madronna in 1976, in conjunction with researchers at Stanford University, compared the safety of homebirth with hospital births. The results showed that morbidity outcomes of the 2,092 births studied were identical. The study also showed that only 5 percent of the mothers birthing at home received medication, whereas 75 percent of the in-hospital births received medication. Even more revealing, three times as many caesarean sections were performed on the mother in hospital births as there were in the planned homebirths that required transfer to a hospital. Babies born in hospitals suffered more foetal distress, newborn infection and birth injuries than did those born in homes. Interestingly, 66 percent of the homebirths were attended by doctors, which would suggest that when women are relaxed in the comfort of their own homes and are allowed to birth normally, what is looked upon as a medical incident can evolve into something quite natural and safe.

Also, not commonly known is that the community midwife who attends homebirths is required to carry the same equipment and drugs that are used to meet the most common special circumstances that occur in hospitals, although their need for it is very rare.

Baby's Choice: Occasionally, while their parents have plans that are quite different, HypnoBirthing babies may decide that it is all right to be born en route to the hospital or even in the comfort of their own homes.

It is important to know that there is nothing about this situation that creates an emergency or that is necessarily cause for panic. As many taxi drivers and policemen will attest, babies can be born safely wherever they choose. Should your baby decide that your bedroom or the backseat of your car, away from the hustle and bustle of other people, is perfectly fine with him, you can remain calm and offer the same gentle birth you had planned earlier.

We suggest that when you set out for the hospital, drape the backseat of your car with plastic bags underneath a sheet, and be sure to bring pillows. It is better to pull over to the side of the road than to risk rushing through traffic. If you are at home, it is better to just get off your feet with something underneath you and relax where you are in your home than to risk having the baby emerge while you're running to get to the car. Baby will be much happier, and you will be better able to maintain the calm and joy of his birthing.

Since much of the apprehension over an unplanned out-of-hospital birth lies in questions about how to handle the umbilical cord, it is important for you to know that leaving the cord attached, even for hours, as is done in some cultures, is safe and quite beneficial to the baby. Your practitioner can offer more details.

A pregnant woman is like a
beautiful flowering tree, but take care
when it comes time for the harvest that you
do not shake or bruise the tree, for in doing so,
you may harm both the tree and its fruit.

Peter Jackson, R.N.

Australia

The Management Styles
of Labour—Compared

T his chapter has been included at the request of parents who expressed a feeling of being well prepared for natural, instinctive birthing, but who felt totally unprepared to meet the protocols that could be imposed in a less-than-natural setting or with a provider who subscribes to Active Management of Labour (AML), and to a lesser degree, even in a standard birth setting.

You can avoid encountering a confrontational situation and/or disappointment if you have prepared thoroughly and discussed these issues with your care provider to determine if the provider is, in fact, on the same page as you are on in regard to gentle birthing. As parents, you need to take responsibility for making choices based on knowledge and questioning. You need to know if the birthing environment and the provider that you are presently with is, in fact, a true fit with your wishes and for how you want the birth of your baby to pay out for mum, baby, and dad.

Management Models

—Active Management of Labour
—Management for Standard or Conventional Birth
—Management for Instinctive-Physiological Birth
—Parental Self-Management for Unassisted Birth

We will explore the various management styles of those care providers who attend births.

Active Management of Labour

• This method of labour involves a concerted effort to forcefully cause the birthing body to do what it already has the innate ability to do with ease, comfort, and dignity if left undisturbed.

• Developed in the late 1960s and 70s in Ireland in an attempt to reduce the number of caesarean sections. It was assumed that mothers who had long labours were traumatised.

• A normal birth, according to AML standards, was about 24 hours. Over the years, that timeline was considerably shortened to 12 hours.

• AML has not decreased the caesarean rate, but instead has had the opposite effect.

• Today, only a few providers in Ireland are becoming more aware of the natural rhythm of birthing and respect that birthing belongs to the family, not to the provider.

Birthing in a hospital does not necessarily mean that your birth will be a managed birth. Some hospitals have gone to great lengths to provide an environment that fits with the goals and wishes of the parents and, not all hospitals, doctors, or midwives engage in Active Management Labour procedures. Many providers refrain from this approach unless circumstances of the birthing deem it necessary in cases of high risk. However, it is sadly true that a very large percentage of hospital facilities and care providers today are needlessly using some, or all, features of AML rather than exercising patience and allowing labour to play out naturally.

If you have chosen a birth attendant who subscribes to AML you are more likely to experience the protocols and interventions that are listed on the management chart that follows this discussion.

Standard or Conventional

The management style that most couples will meet if they choose to birth in a hospital will follow protocols which can be a blend of the regimen of Active Management of Labour and a less strict instinctive physiological labour. Which one of these they encounter depends wholly on the philosophy of the birth attendants. These, too, are listed on the management chart.

Management for Instinctive Birthing

Instinctive births are managed when the need arises. Most care providers who subscribe are happy to honour parents' requests for unmedicated and unintervened births. Parents and medical professionals work together as a team and there is an understanding that should there be a medical indication for intervention, they will have the full cooperation of the parents.

These births are calm, joyful, and peace filled. Babies born in this manner a mellow, content and happy. Parents report that they are easily cared for.

Providers' Management Styles

Active Management of Labour	Standardised Labour
Hospital Setting	**Hospital or Birth Centre**
Physician Managed	Physician/Midwife
Little/No Parent Input	Possible Parent Input
Induction is Scheduled	May/May Not Induce
Early Rupture of Membranes	Release of Membranes
Mandatory IV/Heplock	May Possibly Decline IV
Continuous EF Monitor	Mandatory/Intermittent EFM
Fragmented Labour	Fragmented Labour
Total Food Restriction	Possible Food Restriction
Early Augmentation	Augmentation
Frequent Augmentation	Possible Frequent Augmentation
Chronological Insistence	Some Chronological Expectation
Routine Epidural	Epidural Available
Coached, Forced Pushing	Coached, Forced Pushing
Frequent Infant Heart Decels	Frequent Infant Heart Decels
Use of Oxytocics Post-Birth	Probable Oxytocics Post-Birth
Suctioning of Infant	Probable Suctioning of Infant
Episiotomy is Routine	Infrequent Episiotomy
Immediate Cord Clamping	Probable Immediate Cord Clamping
Land Births Only	Probably Land Births

—A Comparison

Natural, Instinctive Labour	Pure Birth
Free-Standing Centre or Home	**Home Setting**
Midwife/Parent Team	Unassisted
Parents/Provider Team Input	Parents Manage
Spontaneous Onset	Spontaneous Onset
Spontaneous ROM	Spontaneous ROM
No Needle Insertions	No Needle Insertions
Manually Monitored	Self-Monitored
Labour is a Continuum	Labour is a Continuum
Food Allowed	Food Allowed
Natural Augmentation	Natural Augmentation
Augmentation Only as Needed	Augmentation Only as Needed
Clock is Irrelevant	Clock is Irrelevant
No Epidural Use	Natural Relaxation
Body's Natural Expulsive Reflex	Body's Natural Expulsive Reflex
Less Frequent or No Heart Decels	Less Frequent or No Heart Decels
No Oxytocics Used	No Oxytocics Used
Necessary Infant Suctioning Only	Necessary Infant Suctioning Only
Infrequent Episiotomy	No Episiotomy
Delayed Cord Clamping	Delayed Cord Clamping
Water Births and Land Births	Mother's Choice

When Baby Is Breech

In preparation for birthing, sometime between the thirty-second and thirty-seventh weeks of pregnancy, the baby turns from its upright position into what is called a vertex position in preparation for birthing. With this turn, the baby's head is properly positioned down at the mouth of the cervix. Because the head contains the brain and the skull, it is the heaviest part of the baby's body. Once the baby is almost fully developed, the natural pull of gravity is usually sufficient to draw the head down.

Most of the time this turning goes without note, especially if it occurs while the mother is sleeping. The turn can be delayed, however, if the mother is experiencing fear or tension, or if there are circumstances in her life that are upsetting.

Some mothers, for any number of reasons, are reluctant to "let go," and so their uterus remains taut and the baby is not able to complete the turn. When this happens, the baby, deprived of adequate space in which to turn, is unable to complete the rotation and remains in the original, upright position. The baby's buttocks remain at the neck of the uterus in what is called "breech presentation." Sometimes the baby completes only a partial rotation, leaving a shoulder, an arm, or one or both feet positioned at the lower part of the cervix.

A breech position, if not reversed, calls for important decisions. The options are limited to making every effort to help the baby turn, to birth the baby in the breech position, or to resort to a surgical birth. Since few medical providers are trained in the birthing of breech-presented babies, most resort to caesarean births, but this doesn't need to be the first avenue to explore. Many women birth their breech-presented babies vaginally with homebirth midwives.

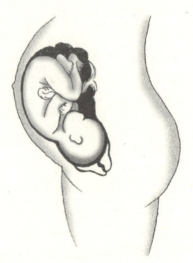

Proper Vertex Position

Helping the Breech-Positioned Baby to Turn

Many babies have been coached to turn with the help of Hypno-Birthing techniques. A special session has proven to be very effective in helping the breech-presented baby to spontaneously reposition into vertex position on its own. This concept is buttressed in a study, presented by Dr. Lewis Mehl-Madronna, formerly of the psychiatric department of the University of Vermont Medical School and Arizona University School of Medicine. The study included 100 women who were referred from practising obstetricians and an additional 100 who responded to an advertisement. Only women who were found to be carrying their babies in breech position at thirty-six weeks gestation or more were included. Mehl-Madronna approached this study looking at reports on serial ultrasound examinations and abdominal palpation that suggested that the likelihood of a breech-positioned baby turning after the thirty-seventh week was no more than 12 percent.

One hundred women in the study group used hypnotherapy. The comparison group consisted of 100 women had no hypnotherapy, though some did have ECV (external cephalic version), a procedure whereby the baby's head is manually manipulated from outside the abdomen to bring about the downward turn.

In the study group, the mothers, while in hypnosis, were led through guided imagery to bring about deep relaxation. Suggestions were then given that they visualise their babies easily turning and see the turn accomplished, with the baby in proper vertex position for birthing. The mothers were helped to visualise the uterus becoming pliable and relaxed in order to allow the baby sufficient room to make the move. The mother was asked to talk to her baby, and the therapists encouraged the baby to release itself from the position it had settled into and to turn downward for an easy birth.

The study ended with 81 of the 100 breech babies in the study group having turned spontaneously from breech position to vertex position. It was originally thought that each mother would require approximately ten hours of hypnotherapy in order to accomplish the desired result.

As the study unfolded, the average number of hours spent with each woman was only four, and half of the successful 81 turns required only one session.

In the comparison group of 100 women who did not participate in hypnotherapy, only 26 babies turned spontaneously. An additional 20 were turned with ECV. It should be noted that it is not uncommon for the baby who is turned through ECV to turn back into breech position. The figures arrived at through this study are considered medically quite significant.

From these findings we see that, in addition to working with visualisation conducive to relaxing the uterus, mothers with babies in breech position can be helped through release therapy. Release therapy is an integral part of the HypnoBirthing programme, where mothers are helped to identify and release negative emotions. If your baby is in breech presentation and there is talk of a possible surgical birth, seek the assistance of your HypnoBirthing practitioner, who will help you with a special hypnosis session that has been found to be especially successful in achieving the desired turn. When the turning of the breech baby is achieved through relaxation and tension release, the baby usually remains in vertex position.

Your practitioner can also help you with finding community resources, acupuncturists, acupressurists, and chiropractors who perform the Webster technique and reflexologists and others who can help with turning techniques. Inquire about "tilting" techniques and other methods for helping the baby to turn. Then, and only then, consider ECV, which is a last resort to avoid a caesarean section. It is not usually a procedure of choice for most women, but it is preferable to surrendering to a surgical birth.

Before Labour:
When Baby Is Ready

From working with HypnoBirthing mothers over many years, I find that our mothers welcome the early signs that labour is near. Sometime prior to term, the mother begins to sense various signals that nature is playing its part in tuning up for the main concert.

Early Signals

Practice Labour: Much talked about but little understood, these surges are nature's way of preparing the uterus for your baby's birthing. They are much like the tightening sensations that are felt during labour, and for that reason we call them practise labour. For first babies, these tightening surges will probably show up sometime during the end of the seventh month. For subsequent pregnancies, they may appear as early as the sixth month.

From day to day you'll experience more of the practise labour surges. As you move and walk, you may even feel a sharp jolt as the pelvic area begins to make room for the baby's journey. This is the pubis bone moving forward and pulling at a ligament here or there. Your body is telling you that it, too, is "getting ready."

Until the final month of pregnancy, these surges are usually erratic and infrequent. As you come near to term, however, you may find that the intervals between them become shorter, and then finally become as frequent as ten- to twenty-minute intervals. Interestingly enough, these surges will sometimes give you a jolt with their pressure like waves, but they are not accompanied by pain. This makes one wonder if the painless pre-labour sensations are further proof of the mind-body connection—the mind knows the body is not ready for labour, so no pain impulse is emitted.

While most people don't consider these surges to be labour, there are many who would disagree and support the belief that the body is already involved in a labour practice that does, in fact, result in the cervix beginning to open. Some mothers will welcome the opportunity to remain relaxed and greet the surges with ease. As you reach term, you will want to take more notice of these sensations so that you don't dismiss what could actually be labour. Many mothers at this time get tuned in to their bodies, and they depend upon this and their instincts to let them know when the real thing has arrived.

Lightening: Several weeks before actual labour begins, the baby "drops" into the lower pelvic area. This is called "lightening." This is usually accompanied by mixed reactions on the part of the mother. It does, indeed, relieve that cramped feeling under the rib cage, and breathing is much easier. However, it also brings about much more pressure on the lower pelvis, and walking becomes a whole new experience. In spite of adjustments that you will have to make for this new position of your baby, you will find, like most other mothers, that your excitement begins to build.

Vaginal Discharge: Occasionally, you may experience more than a slight vaginal discharge that can be clear or whitish. This is another signal that your body is preparing for birth, and it is due to a higher volume of blood flow to that region of your body—another signal that your body is preparing for birth.

Looking at Your "Due Date"

What if your Estimated Due Date (EDD) arrives and labour doesn't start? A whole new set of feelings can spring up. Emotionally and physically, you feel ready "to go"—to birth your baby—but it isn't happening. If you take your due date as gospel and you're not prepared for a possible delay, these days of anticipation can take a toll on you. You may find that anxious, well-meaning family members begin to call regularly to check; your midwife and doctor will begin to take a more watchful eye; fears concerning the baby's well-being can creep in; and each day can start and end with a feeling of disappointment.

Perhaps you'll hear many stories from your friends who chose to be induced when the baby was "overdue." You may even be tempted to accept the subtle suggestions that you don't really need to wait any longer or that "you can be home for the holiday or the weekend." The important thing for you to do is to continue to relax and wait. Your baby knows when it's time to be born. Trust him or her.

Before overreacting to outside pressures, remember that the estimated due date is just that—an estimation. One of our doctors calls it "The Guess Date." Some suggest that it would be more realistic to refer to a birth month or to a segment of the month— "toward the end of September. . ." or "Sometime during the first part of October. . . ."

There are several reasons why your due date is only an estimation. To begin with, the selected date is usually calculated by recalling the date of the first day of your last menstrual period (which may not be accurate), counting back three months from that date and then adding seven days. However, recent studies suggest that for first-time mums, fifteen days should be added, and ten days should be added for mums who have birthed previously.

There are several factors that can skew this estimate: a) Actual calendar months differ in length; b) Menstrual cycles differ in the number of days between periods and in the duration of a period; c) The length of gestation can vary; d) Detection of a heartbeat or foetal movement may seem to support the timely development of the baby at a given point, but it must be remembered that just as children differ in their development, so, too, do babies in utero.

It's interesting to note that the number of babies who arrive on their due date is only around 5 percent, so if your birthing is not "on time," relax. You will be among the 95 percent of parents whose babies are born in advance of the EDD or sometime after the appointed date. The gestation period for 95 percent of normal babies lies within a very broad range of 265 to 300 days from the first day of the mother's last period. The average, taken from those figures, is the 282 days usually used to estimate the due date.

Also interesting is the fact that so many women today are being given as many as three different "due dates" as they proceed through pregnancy. That is certainly an indication that estimates are not solid. How many times did your conception date change?

You need to be able to focus on the fact that the range is between thirty-seven and forty-two weeks. You are not actually "Post Date" until you reach forty-two weeks. Remember, too, that if you are a first-time mother it's not unreasonable to expect that you may go a bit beyond the routine forty-two weeks. Many physicians will not even consider artificial initiation of labour in the absence of any special circumstances until you are at forty-two weeks. Your EDD has no magical significance, and as long as your baby is strong and healthy and you are strong and healthy, don't allow yourself to be pressured into thinking that every day beyond the EDD is a precarious time.

For your baby's sake, resist the temptation to bring medical intervention to your pregnancy when you pass your Guess Date, and certainly don't even consider induction prior to the EDD without a valid medical indication. Induction should occur only when a medical necessity exists for you or your baby. The artificial induction of labour for a baby whose term has been mistakenly calculated could result in birthing a premature baby. It can also mean further medical procedures if your cervix is not "ripe" and ready for birthing.

If it is suggested that you be induced, you owe it to yourself and your baby to have a valid explanation of the reason. You will want to ask about the risks of induction at the time it is recommended, as well as the benefits. Ask to know what your rating is on the "Bishop's Score," which is used to determine the degree to which your body is ready for labour and the probable success of your being induced. Inductions with low Bishop's Scores could mean that the induction could be difficult, leading to lengthy, painful labour and an increased possibility of surgical birth. A score of 8 or 9 would indicate that the induction probably would be successful, but it could also indicate that your baby's birth is near. An induction should be considered only if there is some true medical indication for it.

If you've done a good job initially at securing the support of your caregiver, this should not become a problem for you.

This chart of the Bishop's Score shows the categories that are considered.

Bishop's Score Chart

Cervix		Score		
	0	1	2	3
Position	Posterior	Midposition	Anterior	Anterior
Consistency	Firm	Medium	Soft	Soft
Effacement	0–30%	40–50%	60–70%	80+
Dilation	Closed	1–2 cms	3–4 cms	5 cms+
Station	–3	–2	–1	+1, +2

Neither your body nor your baby understands arbitrary timetables or charts, so take the due date in stride and let Mother Nature and your baby play out their intended roles in their own time. It is the safest and most natural way. Once intervention is introduced in the way of artificial induction, you have already moved away from normal birth. Even the casual suggestion of "just popping that bag" or "doing a little sweep," or helping your labour to start with a "little jump-start," can change the whole ball game for your birthing. These seemingly benign procedures can also result in a labour that is prolonged and sometimes painful if your body is really not "ready to go." When labour is delayed because the cervix is not opening, you may find yourself hearing further suggestions because "Your cervix just doesn't seem to want to open," or your cervix is taking an "inordinate amount of time to get started."

The best advice in looking at your due date is "don't."

Letting Your Baby
and Your Body Set the Pace

Mothers, hold on to your bag of waters.
It is there for a reason.

William and Martha Sears, *The Birth Book*

The actual trigger for the beginning of labour is not entirely known, but it is believed that a hormone secreted from within the baby's body triggers oxytocin, the natural labour-initiating hormone within the mother's body, and the miracle unfolds. That is all part of the master plan—a plan that has a designated flow, but not a designated schedule.

A labour that is slow to start or, later, a resting labour, does not automatically call for the introduction of a chemical stimulant to start or speed up your labour. Nor do these indications necessarily mean a complicated labour. If you experience a latent period when your surges are not starting, or if later the distance between the surges is lengthening, it doesn't mean that your birthing has gone askew. It simply means that the uterus and your baby are not so sure that this is the time yet.

Discussion of rushing in to "jump-start labour" or "move things along" or "augment sluggish surges" can actually bring about the opposite effect and cause a total interruption of the kind of labour that you are planning. If you allow yourself to succumb to these suggestions, you can easily find yourself in the middle of a chemically and chronologically managed labour. If such a comment is made, you or your birthing companion can nicely explain that unless there is a medical urgency, you would like to stay with your birth preferences and that you are in no hurry. One father, when told that if they didn't agree to inducing labour, they could be there all day, commented, "Oh, that's okay. We're not going anywhere." Nature will have its way, and calm is what you need.

Occasionally a mother will find that even when she accepts the suggestion of rupturing her membranes or of using a vaginal gel or Syntocinon drip, her labour still does not move along. Perhaps her body is being prompted into a labour for which it is not quite ready. Since the development of your baby's brain cells is accelerated during the last eight weeks of pregnancy, it seems prudent to let the baby complete this development in utero and not rush birth.

Once artificial induction or augmentation has been introduced in any form, you may find that you have surrendered your choices. Before agreeing to the introduction of procedures or drugs into your body and, therefore, your baby's body, weigh the possibility that you may be placing yourself and your baby on a very slippery slope. Hopefully these issues have weighed heavily upon your decision when you selected your care provider. The birthing room is no place to find that you should have questioned earlier or more often during your pre-natal office visits.

Some women find that by accepting even the smallest doses of synthetic oxytocin, they are able to continue to call on their HypnoBirthing relaxation techniques; others tell us that they tried, but, eventually, Syntocinon won out and they were into even larger doses. They had to request an epidural. This is one of the best reasons for not agreeing to it in the first place unless there is a true medical indication to consider. And, again, we turn to the argument for employing the right caregiver. When the family and caregiver are working together, this discussion will be moot. You will trust that such recommendations will be given only in the event of a situation that genuinely requires a change in the course of your labour.

Few expectant parents really take the time beforehand to explore the risks of deciding to use drugs for faster birth. Parents rarely seek an opportunity to talk with their caregivers about the effects of narcotics upon their pre-born and, subsequently, newborn. No parent would ever choose to give drugs to his or her newborn baby needlessly, but fear of labour can be strong enough to make it simpler for the pregnant family to avoid questions concerning the risks of inductions or epidurals. Similarly, few doctors take the opportunity to explain the adverse side effects of labour drugs with their patients. The matter becomes the medical version of "Don't ask; don't tell."

The well-respected Physicians' Desk Reference (PDR) clearly states that at this time there are no adequate and well-controlled studies for the use of these drugs with pregnant women. The PDR also points out that it is still not known whether these drugs can cause foetal harm when administered to labouring women. There is no hard evidence to support most of these procedures.

Even pills, or any of the injected drugs used to "take the edge off," can suppress a labouring mum's efforts to work with her body's surges, as HypnoBirthing mums are trained to do. An epidural, used to quell the effects of Pitocin/Syntocinon, may offer relief, but it also has a downside. These narcotics can cause reduced muscle tone and prolong labour. Because of the numbing effects of drugs, the labouring woman is less aware of her surges and may not be able to efficiently assist in working with them to facilitate opening. This can prolong labour and often results in increased administration of Pitocin/Syntocinon, leading to continued pain relievers, and so on. A very vicious cycle is established. If she is unable to feel surges and assist in the birthing phase, she could end up with a surgical birth.

Foetology experts are now saying that the disorientation that a baby experiences when his mother has accepted drugs can result in disconnection between mother and baby and cause a long-term feeling of abandonment on the part of the baby. Epidurals, in addition to causing dysfunction in the birthing process, can also cause a woman to run a fever. If this occurs, there is very little remedy except to get the baby born quickly.

If there is talk of induction, turn to the suggested natural means of bringing on labour in the next chapter. Don't dismiss these natural means of initiation, especially professional acupuncture, chiropractic, and acupressure. If you are already in labour, but are being offered augmentation, ask for time to be able to use some of the same natural methods used to initiate labour. Ask for privacy so you can use natural methods—hugs before drugs. As long as indications point to a healthy, strong baby and you are in no danger, be willing to protect your baby from the assault of drugs.

It is important for parents to meet all diagnoses and recommendations with curiosity. They should pause and consider the effects upon the mother and the baby, as well as the overall impact of the birthing experience. It is sometimes difficult for those medical care providers who subscribe to active management of labour to adjust to waiting and "standing by" in the event that they are needed. But if this is how you see your labour advancing and it differs from what you envisioned, you will want to rethink the path that you are on. If you are already beginning to sense that your birthing may go this way, you may want to make some changes now.

When Nature Needs Assistance

While simply going beyond your due date is not by itself cause to bring about medical intervention, on rare occasions a medically risky situation could occur in late pregnancy that should not be brushed aside or ignored as being "nothing." If you experience any of the signals listed below, call your care provider at the earliest possible time. Let your caregiver decide if, indeed, it is nothing or whether your condition requires medical attention.

Such instances include:

- Premature labour (three or more weeks early)

- Diminished foetal motion for more than six hours

- A prolonged period of time from release of the membrane without the natural start of labour

- Persistent and severe headaches—possibly elevated blood pressure

- A strong odour, colour, or significant amount of meconium (greenish-brown, tarlike substance) in the amniotic fluid

- Excessive vaginal bleeding
- Evidence of a prolapsed cord (Get off your feet, raise your buttocks, and call 999.)
- Indication of infection or fever
- Persistent or excessive vomiting or diarrhoea
- Dizziness or blurred vision
- Severe swelling of hands, face, ankles or feet
- Considerably darkened urine
- Unrelenting anxiety over mother's or baby's well-being
- Suicidal thoughts (call 999)

Initiating Labour Naturally

Without these factors, your relaxed attitude can work wonders in bringing about a natural start to your labour along with safe, labour-inducing techniques that you can use naturally and easily:

Hot and spicy foods. Mexican, Indian or Italian foods with "lots of hots" have had more than occasional success in starting labour. By stirring up the digestive processes in your body, you also stir your birthing muscles and your body into action. (Ask your HypnoBirthing practitioner for the special Italian recipe.) This is a good method to combine with any of the other techniques.

Lovemaking (hugs before drugs). If your membrane hasn't released, make love. Semen contains the hormone prostaglandin, which helps to soften the cervix. Here we see nature going full circle—what entered the uterus to help make the baby can help get it out. Kissing, hugging, fondling, and gentle finger or oral nipple or clitoral stimulation triggers the hormonal connection between the breast and vagina, producing the natural oxytocin that can start uterine surges. It is helpful to bring the mother to orgasm. If the stimulation of one nipple is not sufficient to start surges, try stimulation of both nipples simultaneously. However, prolonged or vigorous nipple stimulation of both nipples is not advised as it can have an adverse effect on your baby by creating hyperstimulation.

Visualisation. While your nipple or clitoris is being stimulated, use the rosebud visualisation, focusing on the rosebud's slowly unfolding and opening. Gently direct your breath down into the vaginal region while visualising.

Walk. Walk, walk, and then walk some more.

Bath. A medium-hot bath often provides the relaxation you need. You or your partner can scoop the water over your nipples and your abdomen. Take a shower, directing the hot water over your abdomen.

Fear release. Have your birth companion take you through a fear-release session similar to the one practised in class so that you can search your thoughts to see if there are any lingering fears, emotions, or unresolved issues that you need to release. Locked-up emotions can make you feel uptight and cause your body to produce inhibiting catecholamine. Your tension can translate into a tense cervix, preventing the flow of your natural relaxants. If you feel you need professional help, call your HypnoBirthing instructor for an individual fear-release session or ask for a referral to a hypnotherapist. It works wonders. Use this time for talking to the baby.

Acupressure. An acupressurist can facilitate the natural onset of labour almost immediately and yet afford you the time to make whatever preparations you need. Using the services of a professional will improve your chances of having the most effective points used and of obtaining faster results. It can also be helpful for use during labour. Do not apply pressure to these points other than at a time when you are ready to initiate labour.

Acupuncture/auricular therapy. Like acupressure, there are points that an acupuncturist or an auricular therapist can activate for the easy and effective induction of labour. These are relatively easy procedures and offer a much smoother entry into labour. Like the acupressure points, it is important that these points not be stimulated during pregnancy except for the purpose of induction when labour is slow to start or during a labour that has slowed.

Seeking the services of homeopathic and naturopathic doctors can be beneficial in collaboration with the recommendation above when these other recommendations have not been sufficient.

When you have exhausted all these means of natural initiations of labour, and it is determined that artificial induction by Pitocin/Syntocinon drip is an absolute necessity, you may request that only a minimal dose be administered and that it not be increased without your consent. You will also want to ask that the Pitocin/Syntocinon be withdrawn once your body has taken over. Many of our mothers report that the HypnoBirthing relaxation techniques that they mastered saw them through even with an induced labour, but it should be a last resort.

The Onset of Labour

L abour is usually defined as that period from the time that your cervix actually begins to thin and open until the moment that the baby is born.

HypnoBirthing recognises only two phases of labour: the Thinning and Opening Phase, and then the actual Birthing Phase, where the baby descends as his mother assists with Birth Breathing.

For the purpose of this study, I am covering in this chapter the more familiar aspects of labour as experienced by most couples. Much of the material applies to most birthing women whether they are birthing in a hospital setting, free-standing birth centre, or in their homes.

Labour will start with the first phase anytime between 37 and 42 weeks of pregnancy. The 40-week estimation of term is called EDD (Estimated Due Date). From 40 weeks, gestation period is expressed as 40.1; 40.2; 40.3; and so on. First-time mums average a gestation period of 41.3. A woman is not post date, or late, until she has reached 42.0.

The most common signs of the onset of labour are:

The release of the membranes (can be leaking or a sizeable gush).

Release of the uterine seal and birth show.

Uterine surges often up to 30 minutes apart.

A feeling of constipation or loose stooling.

Surges that form a pattern.

None of the above (some women report only tightness around the abdominal area).

Sometimes the release of membrane is an early sign of labour; for others, it may not occur until just before the baby is born. Babies can even be born "en caul," with the membrane surrounding them like a veil.

If the release of your membranes is the first signal that your labour is beginning, you will want to check the fluid to be sure that it:

1. is clear with no particles, except for an occasional show of white vernix, the cheeselike covering that surrounds the baby in the sac;

2. has no colour;

3. has no putrid odour.

When the membranes release, call your care provider to report that you have examined the fluid, and it meets all of the conditions mentioned above. Assure the caregiver that you wish to remain at home until your labour is under way and that you will call before leaving for the hospital. If you have hired the right caregiver, this should be the end of the conversation.

You may begin to hear of the danger of infection. This often is followed by the suggestion that you come into the hospital "to be checked" so that antibiotics can be administered to prevent infection or so that you can be monitored. While infection is a possibility, it is a very rare one, and it is not imminent. Bacteria have to be introduced into the body in order for infection to take place. As one doctor says, "The vagina is not a straw." Another advises, "The vagina is not a sponge." When you step out of the bathtub, there is no flow of water that has gathered in the vagina. One of our doctors reminds his mothers that bacteria are not sperm, and they don't swim. Don't be intimidated by talk of early infection if there is no indication of infection.

Accepting a vaginal exam can be the first step toward artificial induction. Often being checked translates to "check-in," followed by pressure to jump-start your labour. If you remain at home until your labour really starts, you will avoid both of these interventions.

Sometimes there is a considerable delay between the time that your membrane releases and active labour starts. This doesn't mean that something is wrong. In the event that the onset of labour is delayed, refer back to the suggestions for initiating labour naturally. Don't buy into the notion that labour must be started immediately. Chances are, labour will start on its own within twenty-four hours. Buy time and request that you wait for another couple of hours or so. Your temperature can be monitored. If your labour is delayed for a long period of time, and you are being pressured to have your labour induced, request that antibiotics be administered. Politely decline any vaginal exams. It's that simple. It is not necessary that an induction procedure be initiated, barring any other indications of a need to do so. Agreeing to that first intervention or to an artificial induction in the absence of medical indication could turn your plans for a calm birth upside down.

You will know that the onset of true labour has arrived when you experience uterine surges that are rhythmic—tightening and releasing in a distinct pattern. You may or may not feel your uterine surges starting. Some mothers report feeling only a tightening sensation in and around the abdomen at the onset of their labour. For many HypnoBirthing mothers, these sensations are not accompanied by discomfort. They are not convinced that their labour has actually begun. Some report only that they feel constipated and need to relieve their bowels.

Before or after you experience your first uterine surge, you may discover that the uterine seal that prevents bacteria from entering the uterus has dislodged. "This birth show" is a stringy discharge that can be clear, tinged, slightly pink, or bright red.

From the time you were admitted at the hospital or birthing centre, your assessment will be judged by how long you have been in labour. Don't allow yourself or your birth companion to become overly caught up in the mechanics of timing and charting. You will sense when the intervals between surges are becoming shorter if you listen to your body frequently.

The months of conditioning and practice are now paying off. Your positive attitude and confidence will allow you to remain calm and relaxed.

When your surges begin, use relaxation and Slow Breathing to increase the efficiency of each surge, visualising the opening rosebud and breathing gently down toward your vagina. This will encourage the uterus to start surging.

The calm HypnoBirthing approach to birth inhibits secretion of catecholamines, so it is likely that your digestive functioning will not be arrested. You need energy and you need to snack; drink lots of fluids to avoid dehydration and keep your bladder empty.

At your signal—usually closing your eyes—your birth companion will know that you are in surge and will stroke your arm while reciting the cues that are on the Birth Companion's Prompt Card (available from your HypnoBirthing instructor). It's not necessary to follow the prompts line by line. These are suggestions for the kinds of phrases that will assist you in remaining relaxed.

The most important factor to consider during labour may be what you sense and feel, not what you see or hear. As your birth companion gives prompts, trust your body and go deeper within each surge that you breathe up, maximising each surge to the fullest. Trust your body, as it knows and will tell you when it is the best time to move to a birthing facility. If you are birthing at home, continue to relax and stay at home.

The illustration that follows shows a comfortable birthing mother lying in a lateral position during labour.

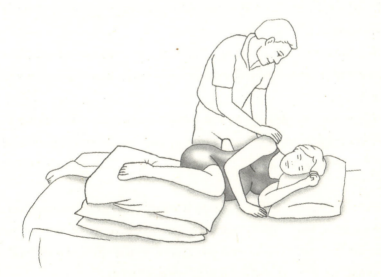

Lateral Position During Labour

As Labour Advances: Thinning and Opening

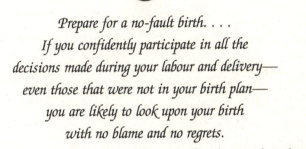

Prepare for a no-fault birth. . . .
If you confidently participate in all the
decisions made during your labour and delivery—
even those that were not in your birth plan—
you are likely to look upon your birth
with no blame and no regrets.

William Sears and Martha Sears, *The Birth Book*

A s you move through the Thinning and Opening Phase of your labour, you will find that your many weeks of preparation are now stepping in to assist you as you turn your birthing over to your baby and your body. You call upon your natural birthing instinct and literally "do nothing" but allow your body to remain loose and limp. Creating a nest, as you did when you practised, can greatly assist you in reaching a wonderful feeling of lightness and buoyancy. Nesting is illustrated earlier in this book.

Instead of looking upon your labour in fragments, as is the case in most other programmes, you will see your labour as a continuum. You may hear mention of centimeters and discussion of how "open" your cervix is. Pay no attention to those numbers. HypnoBirthing mothers blow those figures right out of the water. One can be at only four centimeters at one vaginal exam and, surprisingly, at seven or eight at the next exam. The number tells you little or nothing, and certainly they are not a valid gauge of how long your labour will last. They tell you only where you are at that given moment. Relax and just visualise the cervix opening in a continuing manner, as shown in the illustration.

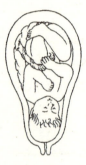 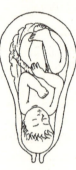

Not thinned   **2 cms.**   **5 cms.**   **Complete**
or opened   **opened**   **opened**

Hallmarks of Labour

During this period, you will probably experience at least one or more of the hallmarks of labour—those milestones that tell you that your labour is moving along. They are all very natural and good messages from your body. Your birth companion will remind you of the hallmarks as you pass each one. It's exciting.

- Your body heat will rise and/or drop alternately. One minute you will be kicking off bedding; in another you'll be requesting a warmed blanket.

- When you get up to empty your bladder, there may be a spot of blood on your sanitary pad. The body is directing its efforts downward.

- You may begin to hiccup, burp, feel nauseated, or even vomit as your diaphragm has an initial reaction to the lower pulsations in your body that will soon move your baby down to birth. The good news is that it doesn't last long. (It happens rarely with HypnoBirthing mums because their bodies are calm and not in tumult.)

- Regardless of how calmly and well you have approached your birthing, you may all of a sudden feel the need "to escape." Even a mum who is having a fantastic birthing has been known to express the thought, "I don't think I want to do this any longer" or "I can't do this anymore." This last hallmark is one of the most exciting. It means that the birth of your baby is right around the corner. Your birth companion will remind you of this hallmark, and the mood changes for everyone in the room. Your baby is almost here.

What Is Happening?

The cervix is thinning. The longitudinal fibres of the uterus continue to draw back the circular fibres so that the cervix increasingly thins and opens.

You will continue to experience the wave of each surge. Your abdomen will feel as though it is surging upward, tightening, and then receding back down again. These surges usually last no more than thirty-five to forty-five seconds at this point. Keeping your body limp and relaxed allows this stage to pass with little or no discomfort. Intervals between surges can vary considerably.

Clutching, clenching, or curling up in a foetal position all create tension in your body that is counterproductive. You will also want to avoid getting caught up in activities and options that hospital staff will offer with kind intentions (unless those activities or options appeal to you). Mothers frequently say that suggestions that they take walks, spend time in a rocker, or "get things moving" distracted them and broke their deep level of relaxation.

You will hear that your muscles will work more efficiently if you walk and remain active. In 1997 a study in Texas, conducted through the University of Texas Southwestern Medical Centre, found that there were no significant differences between the length of labour of women who walked and those who remained sitting, relaxing, or resting. I have never observed animal mothers walking halls. Instead, they seem to go deeper into relaxation.

HypnoBirthing mothers find that their cervixes seem to open more easily and quickly as a result of giving those muscles the necessary relaxation and oxygenated blood flow needed to open.

If you feel that you would like to walk, then do so, but not because you are being pressured to get on your feet and get those muscles moving.

Attempting to overcome or manipulate labour can cause fatigue and discouragement. If you have spent a sufficient amount of time conditioning your mind and body, the art will be there for you. Follow the techniques that you learned, and trust in yourself and your body's ability to birth. You'll be fresh, alert, and fully energised when that wonderful moment of birth arrives.

"Tubbers"

I spoke to a labour and birthing nurse recently who couldn't rave enough about how successful her "tubbers" were at combining HypnoBirthing and water birthing. We are seeing many women choose the comfort and ease of water birthing. It is an extraordinarily good complement to HypnoBirthing, enhancing your relaxation and allowing the baby to be born into an environment that makes for an easy transition from life within the womb to air breathing. There is no doubt about the merit of the weightlessness and buoyancy that water provides. When women use this combination, their minds are free and relaxed, and their bodies are better able to benefit from the softening effect that water has on the birthing muscles and on the folds of the perineum. One therapy contributes to the efficacy of the other.

The association between water and sensuality is also not wasted on couples who are birthing. That's because it is understood that water gives us a feeling of pleasure, contentment, and well-being. Water will help this phase of labour pass in a way that is beyond comparison.

Slow or Resting Labour

I t is not uncommon for a labour to slow, then to accelerate, slow again, and then reach completion. The best way to manage a slowed or resting labour is to meet it with patience. The one thing you don't want to see happening is that you succumb to the notion that this is a trouble sign and the labour must be augmented. Most HypnoBirthing families are better able to get through this without intervention because they do not have continual Electronic Foetal Monitor (EFM).

Introduced onto the birthing scene in the 1980s, these machines were devised to help monitor the labours of women who were high-risk; but now with one in every room, the devices have become a huge drawback for the family who is not at risk. The biggest drawback of having an EFM in the birthing environment is that some medical care-givers tend to get overly caught up with tracings and patterns. There is the mistaken belief that a woman's cervix must open according to some regulated pattern or time frame, or it needs to be "fixed." The baby often ends up on the short end of the fixing.

A resting labour later does not mean that immediate steps need to be taken to restart the labour. Nature will have its way, and calm is what you need. After experiencing the calm of a nap, many mothers resume an active and even accelerated labour.

If you should experience a slow or resting labour, ask for time to be able to use some of the same natural methods used to initiate or restart a resting labour. Ask for privacy so you can use natural methods—hugs before drugs. As long as you and your baby are healthy and strong, and you are in no danger, be willing to protect your baby from the assault of drugs.

Occasionally, when a mother accepts the suggestion of rupturing her membranes or of using a Syntocinon drip, her labour does not move along more rapidly.

Unless it's a true medical urgency, the family should pause and consider the effects of any intervention upon the mother and the baby, as well as the overall impact of the birthing experience.

In addition to employing some of the suggestions in the section on inducing labour naturally, there are several ways in which you can pass time during a slow or resting labour that actually enhance your comfort and contribute to the opening and spreading of the pelvic area. For example:

The Birth Ball: The birth ball serves many purposes: It can offer you an alternative to remaining in bed during a prolonged labour; it is an excellent prop for you to support yourself by the side of your bed while your birthing companion applies Light Touch Massage; and it relaxes the pelvic muscles. Many hospitals provide birth balls for labouring mothers. Feel free to request one or bring your own. They're fun and so beneficial.

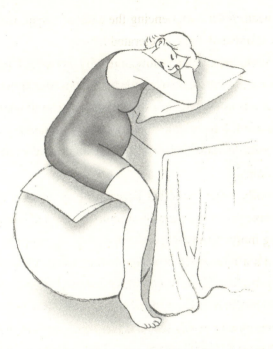

Labouring Mother Resting on a Birth Ball

Bath or Birth Pool: The benefits of the bath or birth pool have already been explained. Many mothers delight in spending a good deal of time in them if their labours are taking time. In order to derive the most benefit from your stint in the bath, place a towel from the tips of your nipples down to your thighs to keep the protruding parts of your body warm. While gently scooping water over your body, your birthing companion can recite the usual prompts during your surges.

Shower: A warm shower, with the water directed to your abdomen, is also a good way to pass time and gives the effect of effleurage.

Humour: The breathing produced by laughter is one of the best means of relaxing. Pack several pieces of humourous reading. Humour

increases the production of endorphins, which, in turn, block the introduction of catecholamine.

Nipple Stimulation: The stimulation of one or both nipples triggers
the hormonal connection between the breast and the vagina, producing
your body's natural oxytocin that can enhance your uterine surges.
Ask for the privacy to be able to use nipple stimulation. Your medical
caregivers will be neither surprised nor embarrassed at your request.

If Labour Weakens

There may come a time when all accommodation to your wishes has
been extended, but, for some reason, an obvious pattern of decreased
or severely weakened uterine activity forms; and your baby is not
weathering it well. In such an instance, it may be determined that your
birthing needs medical assistance.

In this kind of situation, you will find that being a part of the
decision-making team will help you accede to whatever preparations
need to be made. You will remain calm and in control of your circumstances. This is HypnoBirthing.

Nearing Completion

You are reaching the end of the Thinning and Opening Phase. Your surges are closer, stronger, and more beneficial. The wall of your cervix has completely thinned, and the cervix is continuing to open sufficiently to allow the baby to begin to move down. When this happens, your body sends a message that it's time to change from Slow Breathing to Birth Breathing—the gentle, but firm, breathing down that will help you to bypass lengthy, difficult, and fatiguing "pushing" techniques used by other methods.

Time distortion usually sets in, and you lose track of time. You will be more aware of the working of your uterus, with waves rising almost as though your birthing body is separate from the rest of your body; you may or may not be aware that the surges are becoming longer and higher. As you breathe each one up to the fullest, they become more efficient. The touch and voice of your birth companion will guide you through each surge. Your journey becomes more encouraging, as labour from this point can move along very quickly, especially as you deepen your relaxation.

You drift into an almost amnesiac state, focusing on your birthing experience. You will find that conversations in the room become fuzzy; and even if you are spoken to, it just seems like almost too much effort to respond. You go deeper and deeper, and your mind relaxes and rests. At this point you are fully birthing instinctively. You just get out of the way and let your body do the work. At the end of this phase, as your cervix becomes fully opened, you will feel the fullness within your body and, unless you experience a resting time, you will instinctively feel the need to change your breathing pattern to the downward Birth Breathing to assist the baby in his descent. It is essential that you understand that from this point on there is no pathological reason for discomfort, unless you allow yourself to slip out of this amnesiac state and assume the tension within your body.

During this time your body assists you with its natural expulsive reflex (NER). It is important more than ever that you do nothing and allow your body to do its job of taking charge of your baby's descent. To help you further, the vaginal wall becomes lubricated and expands. The rhythmic pulsations move the baby down.

What Feelings You May Experience

Your mood will remain calm and nearly euphoric. You may go through this final phase of opening in an almost dreamlike state. Nature's amnesia will lull you so that you seem to drift in and out of alertness. It becomes even easier to place your awareness only on your baby and your birthing body.

As time distortion clicks in, the length of the surge will be distorted, and your time consciousness will fade. Twenty minutes will, indeed, seem like five. This is nature's way of helping you remain placid and serene. At the end of this phase, your shift to Birth Breathing will give you a feeling of well-being, as you and your baby work together.

How You May Participate

At this time, you really settle into birthing. Your conversant stage has passed, and you are easing into the business of having a baby. Deep relaxation and a thoroughly limp body help you to block out your surroundings and go even further within to your baby.

By this time, many women have already adopted a lateral position. If you choose to stay on your back, your birthing companion needs to be sure that the head of the bed is elevated so that you are not lying flat. Lying flat can limit the supply of oxygen to your baby. Your birthing companion will help you to adjust your position if you slip down in the bed.

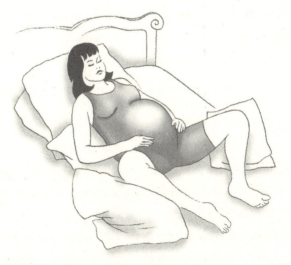

Semi-Reclining Position Modified

With deepened relaxation, you let go and let your baby and your body do what each can do best during this time. You will continue to breathe up with your uterine surges until your cervix opens, but it will seem almost effortless. With the signal of downward lower fullness, you will know instinctively that it is time to change your breathing to Birth Breathing. Your birth companion will assure staff that you are not going to push at this point; and it is safe for you to change to a Birth Breath.

With no effort, you move closer to a place of utter comfort, moving in harmony with your body.

When your body sends the message that it is time to begin to nudge your baby down, you will follow the lead of your body and work with the shift of your pulsations that now direct your breathing downward in contrast to the upward breathing that you have been doing up until now. Often this is all accomplished with little notice; you continue to work with your surges quietly and serenely without changing position.

You should not be alone, even though you may appear to be perfectly relaxed and simply resting. That look can be deceiving, as few others are aware that you are breathing your baby down to the vaginal outlet.

The Pelvic Station

The location of the baby's head within the pelvic region is measured by what is known as the Pelvic Station. You will hear reference to the Pelvic Station both before and during your birthing. As the baby journeys downward, his progress may be explained to you as being at -1 or +1 or +2. Positive numbers are below the midsection of the pelvis; negative numbers are above the midsection. The measure is determined by where the "presenting part" or top of the baby's head is. If you are told that the head is high, it means that the position is still in the minus level. The head is said to be engaged when the head is at 0.

The Pelvic Station

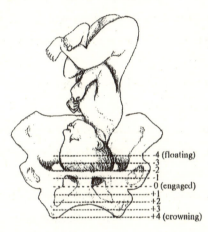

-4 (floating)
-3
-2
-1
0 (engaged)
+1
+2
+3
+4 (crowning)

Every child is unique. Every child must
pass through the same stages, leading from an
enclosed world to the open one, from being
folded in on itself to reaching outward.

Frederick Leboyer, M.D., *Birth Without Violence*

Practice Positions
Also Used in Birthing

What Is Happening?

What is happening is **birth**! Your baby gradually descends to the rim of the perineum, and the baby's head becomes visible (crowning). With the head nearly or fully crowned, you are ready now to give those final few breaths that will bring the baby past the perineal rim and into the world. After birth, your baby is placed immediately on the skin of your abdomen or lower chest for embrace and bonding with you and your birth companion. When the umbilical cord stops pulsating, the cord will be cut, and you, your baby, and your birthing companion continue to bond.

The more nature is able to take its course, the less likely you are to need an episiotomy. In the same way that the neck of the cervix needed to be gradually thinned and opened, the thick rim of the perineum needs to gradually thin and unfold through each surge by natural pressure of the baby's head until, at last, the folds open fully to allow the baby's head to pass through. It appears to be a slow unraveling, but, to the contrary, it is more swiftly accomplished with Birth Breathing than by any other means. HypnoBirthing mums talk of three or four Birth Breaths to bring the baby past the perineum and out.

Birth Breathing is the opposite of Slow Breathing, where you drew the surge up and worked with the upward wave. Now, instead of breathing up, you will take in a short, deep breath and breathe down. Your birthing companion will prompt you to direct your breath and love downward to help your baby move smoothly down to crowning. As you exhale, breathe down and visualise the opening of your vagina like the petals of a rose, folding outward as your baby moves to the perineal rim.

If the move is going smoothly, you may choose to remain in a lateral position (see illustration to follow) and simply breathe down until the baby's head is visible, or you may wish to adopt the Slanted "J" position, being sure to rest just above your tailbone to allow the baby plenty of room to move out. If your baby needs some help in moving down smoothly, you may want to adopt some of the positions that are described and illustrated in the following pages. Some of the recommended positions are designed to help the muscles and pelvic structure to spread and open more freely. Many of the positions call for your birth companion to assist you so that the two of you can take part in your baby's birth together.

Toilet Sitting Position

This position that you have been using throughout your pregnancy on a daily basis will also prove to be a very comfortable one to alternate with other positions during your birthing

Many women find a great deal of comfort in Toilet Sitting while they are still in the opening phase and while breathing their baby down.

The body naturally responds to this position as it is conditioned to release and let go when toileting. The two sets of muscles are closely related, and the Natural Expulsive Reflex (NER) present in birthing is supported by Birth Breathing. This position can offer the kind of spread that helps your pelvic area, opens your vagina, utilises gravity, and relieves you from having to support yourself on your legs. Just place a pillow or two behind your back and relax. As you near the crowning period, you will have to assume another of the birthing positions in order to safely birth your baby.

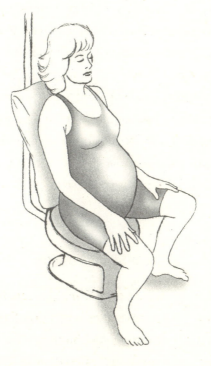

Toilet Sitting

Additional Relaxation and Birthing Positions

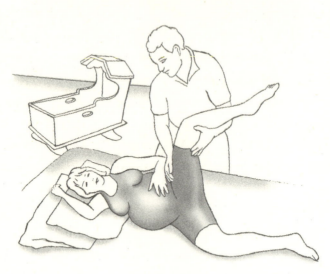

Lateral Position

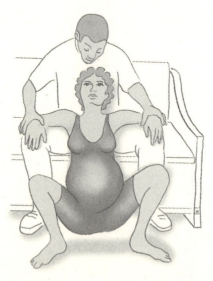

Companion Supported Squat Position

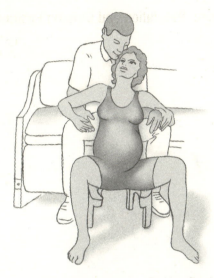

Supported Position on Birthing Stool

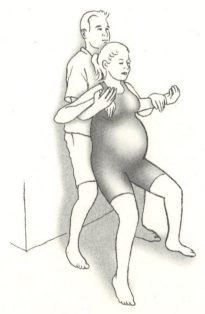

Companion Supported Upright Position

These are additional positions to use during the birthing stage that can be adopted by the birthing mother without the assistance of her companion. They are as follows:

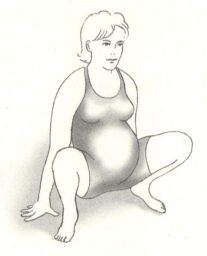

Leaping Frog Positions

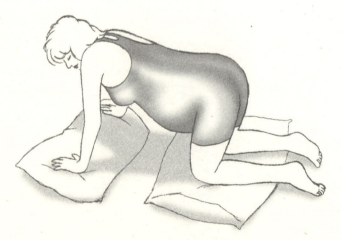

Hands-and-Knees Position

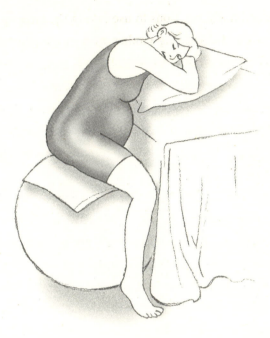

The Birth Ball

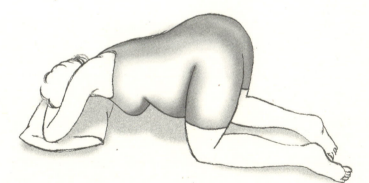

Polar Bear Position

Polar Bear: While the Polar Bear position is not a birthing position, it can be helpful if the baby is found to be in a less than optimal
position for emergence. This favourable position can be assumed from
a Hands-and-Knees position by placing your forearms on the floor in
front of you and resting your forehead on your hands. Both the Polar
Bear and the Hands-and-Knees position allow your baby to move back
from the lower pelvic area and turn to a more beneficial position for
birthing if this is needed.

If the baby does need an assist to move to a more optimal position,
the Rebozo technique can be nicely utilised while mother is in the
Polar Bear position. The technique, developed by midwife Guadalupe
Trueba, is well known in Mexico and is fast making its way into birthing rooms in the United States. It is simply done by placing a long
scarf under the mother's abdomen at the area of the pelvic region and
lifting upward. This manoeuvre lifts the baby out of the present position and provides her with an opportunity to, in effect, back up and
return to the birth path in a more favourable position for easy birthing.

Your Baby Crowns and Births

This is the first time that you "see" the results of your labour as the tip of the baby's head becomes visible. You will feel encouraged when you reach this point. The natural pulsations of your body will slowly urge your baby forward as you continue to direct the breathing that assists your baby to crowning.

When the top of the head is fully visible, one or two more surges are usually all that are needed to gently birth the baby's head. It is amazing how easily a head can pass through the elastic-like perineum if you remain relaxed. Tears in the skin can be avoided if the mother has practised perineal massage and there are no rushed, violent pushes.

The birth companion will continue to help you return to a relaxed state between surges. Birthing prompts are repeated here also. The entire pelvic area should be kept as relaxed as possible. Directing your breath toward the vagina and helping the baby to move forward will help the perineum to unfold.

If everything is fine, the baby should be birthed fully before suctioning or other routines are performed, and one of the parents should receive the baby if that is their wish. The handling of the baby by someone other than a parent should be minimal and utilised only if necessary. This will help make the baby's transition into her new surroundings less traumatic. Many caregivers now are happy to assist a parent in this.

Bonding

If you don't already know if your baby is a boy or a girl, you'll not have to wait long, for as soon as the baby is born, your birthing companion will announce the sex of the baby to you. You'll share this happy time together while caregivers visibly observe the baby's condition and assess mum's needs.

The baby is placed immediately on your bare chest or abdomen for bonding. Remarkably, studies called Kangaroo Mother Care, out of Australia, have found that the mother's body heat adjusts to the needs of her newborn.

At this point the birthing companion places his hand on the baby's back to offer the security of skin-to-skin bonding that is so important during these first few moments. Handling by others should be minimal, if not absent entirely. The baby needs to feel safe among the people whose scents and energies she is most familiar with.

There is no need to rush to "clean" the baby, nor to cut the cord. It is more important for the newborn to experience skin contact with both of its parents, if possible. The vernix caseosa, that cheesy covering that makes your baby look like a channel swimmer, will simply be absorbed into the baby's skin—it is a gift from nature. Any excesses will be removed later when baby has her first bath.

You will experience exhilaration beyond compare in these first few incredible moments as you and your birth companion touch and hold the baby, watching her begin to stretch and move and unfold, gaining a tactile sense of her new environment, one arm and one leg at a time.

Bonding during those first few precious moments of your baby's life will provide a natural high that defies description, and the feeling that you and your companion experience will remain with you for the rest of your lives. This is when the relationship that began before your baby was born is reaffirmed with actual skin-to-skin bonding—mother and father and baby (or other birthing companion) embracing in loving union.

It is during this time that a loving relationship is affirmed, and this wonderful happening should not be rushed. Through your caresses, gaze, and soft conversation, you validate your infant's acceptance and approval. The baby feels this love, and her feelings of security and self-worth are validated.

HypnoBirthing practitioners who have witnessed that first gaze when the infant's eyes meet with his parents' cite this as one of the most spiritual times in their lives as birthing educators.

Like all mammals, babies are genetically and instinctively programmed to take to the breast. You may wish to bond with your baby in this way, while the birth companion continues to support the baby's body with his hand or becomes involved with the cutting of the cord. Allowing your baby to complete the crawl to the breast has physical, as well as psychological, benefits. This contact and stimulation at the breast causes your uterus to begin to contract, helps to expel the placenta, and appropriately closes blood vessels to avoid any possible excessive bleeding. Your midwife will offer suggestions and assistance to help you and your baby as you experience your first feeding.

More is written on the importance of secluding yourselves with your baby to help her adjust to this new earthly environment in the chapter "Birth Afterglow."

Baby Is Born

You should be informed of the first appearances of your baby's head in a calm manner. There is a tendency for those in attendance to begin to direct this phase with loud, animated cheers. I stress that birthing is not an athletic event. Voices should not be raised. This is as much for your baby as for you. Your baby hears every sound; the sounds that he hears should not frighten him.

What You Will Feel

There is no need for discomfort during the birthing phase of labour. The cervix has already thinned and opened, and now the gradual descent of the baby is conducted in such a way that there is no strain on the tissues and sphincters of the birth path. Movies and television notwithstanding, if this descent is completed as you have practised, there is no reason for pain or any other sensation. Most women experience this birthing phase calmly as they breathe down and ultimately help the baby to emerge. There is no doubt that this is the most beautiful time of birthing. This is the culmination of everything you've planned and waited for during the last nine months.

Birth Breathing

For a good portion of the birthing phase, your body and baby will be working in harmony, as the natural expulsive reflex (NER) takes over and moves your baby down the birth path. You will assist by using the breathing technique that you have been practising for some time. Once your baby's head becomes visible, you will continue to use this downward nudge breath until the baby is gently breathed past the opening folds of the perineum and emerges in birth.

This phase cannot be taken lightly if you wish to birth easily and efficiently. Just as you needed to practise Surge Breathing to bring yourself past the thinning and opening phase, you will need to practise Birth Breathing. While in labour, you will follow your body's lead and work with it when you feel the onset of a surge. Here are some helpful hints:

- The best place to practise this breathing style is on the toilet as you are moving your bowels. Become aware of the pulsations that move the stool down and out. Your breaths are short intakes with gentle nudging breaths downward—nothing forceful. Practising in this way will show you that it actually accomplishes the task more easily and quickly.

- Your eyes may remain closed if you choose to stay in deep relaxation through this period. Since you will not be forcefully pushing, there is no need for you to keep your eyes open to avoid tearing the tiny blood vessels in your eyes.

- Placing the tip of your tongue at the place where your front teeth and palate meet will help your lower jaw to recede so that you remain free of tension in your mouth and jaw area. This will also help to relax the vaginal outlet.

- When you feel the onset of a surge, follow it. Take in a short, but deep, breath through your nose and direct the energy of that breath to the lower back of your throat and down through your body behind your baby in the form of a "J"—down and forward. Allow all the muscles in your vaginal area to open as though you were letting the breath out through them or moving your bowels. Don't ride out or hang on to a breath beyond its effectiveness; and don't allow those lower muscles to tighten.

- Repeat this process by taking in another short, deep breath and breathe down in the same pattern as above—and then another.

- Repeat this motion several times with each surge as your body leads you through this part of birthing your baby down to crowning. Continue to work with your body as long as it is still surging. Breathing down only once during a surge can cause you to lose the effectiveness of the surge, prolong the birthing time, and waste your energy.

- Firmly direct your breathing down through your body. Don't let the thrust of your breath escape through your mouth. These are not shallow breaths, but they are also not strenuous. These are deep breaths, with the energy of the breath going right down to your vagina.

- You may experience the sensation of needing to move your bowels, and that is exactly the region to which you need to direct the thrust of your breath. That is the reason we ask you to practise on the toilet.

• With the exhalation of each breath, your birthing companion will prompt you to breathe love and energy down to your baby, to open the path and to nudge your baby down to birth.

Your baby is now ready to come out and must be allowed to come easily. The head births first; the vulva gradually distends without discomfort; the baby's body emerges, often requiring only more gentle bearing down.

Many HypnoBirthing mothers who have thoroughly mastered relaxation and deepening techniques are surprised to learn that none of the steps described above are necessary. A relaxed body can actually propel the baby through the path to emergence on its own.

Post-Birth Activities

Still at work for you, your body reacts to the euphoria you are feeling by stimulating the uterus into the final stage. The umbilical cord is cut after it stops pulsating. With one or two more surges, the placenta is born. You and your birth companion bond with your new baby.

From this point on, all who share this wonderful miracle experience a very enjoyable high. Often doctors and midwives who witness HypnoBirthing express awe at participating in the experience. An indefinable feeling of joy and pleasure sweeps in and takes over. You and your birthing companion may be oblivious to the activities of medical caregivers at this point as you experience getting acquainted with your new baby.

It is important that the clamping and cutting of the cord be delayed until after it stops pulsating. When the cord is prematurely cut, it abruptly cuts off the flow of blood to the baby, depriving him of that source of oxygen and of the many nutrients that will affect his health for a lifetime. Allowing the baby to take his first breaths with the continued benefit of oxygen from the placenta eases the task of taking air into his lungs once he is outside the womb. It is an easier and more comfortable introduction to breathing.

Your baby is put to the breast. HypnoBirthing babies, alert and comfortable, usually take to the breast within minutes of their birth.

Dr. Lennart Righard's Delivery Self-Attachment video, resulting from a study in Denmark published in 1990, shows the ability of newborns who were not medicated during labour to crawl to the mother's breast, just as other mammals do, and suckle. On the other hand, even with help, the babies whose mothers were medicated lacked the ability to crawl to the breast and were unable to suckle even with assistance.

When the cord has stopped pulsating, it is clamped. Your companion, if he or she chooses, may take part in cutting the cord, separating the baby from the cord and placenta.

The expulsion of the placenta should be allowed to occur naturally with just one or two pushes as your uterus continues to surge. You may or may not be aware of these continued surges as your placenta is birthed. These final surges help your placenta to loosen from the wall of the uterus and assist the uterus to begin to assume its normal size. Allowing your placenta to break away in this normal manner can take anywhere from five to thirty minutes. In the event that the placenta is not birthed within a reasonable amount of time, your medical caregiver may suggest a medical assist. The cord should not be pulled in order to effect an extraction.

Your midwife or doctor will examine your placenta and then the abdomen to determine the "status" of your uterus.

An indescribable feeling of joy, excitement, and even giddiness sweeps in and takes over. Congratulations! Your miracle is complete.

Breastfeeding Is Best Feeding

Contributed by Robin Frees,
Lactation Consultant, HypnoBirthing practitioner

I t is your baby's "birth" day. If you could ask your baby about the best gift he could get from you, what would that be? Your baby would want to breastfeed. So before making a decision about infant feeding, consider the following thoughts and information. Give breastfeeding a try; and make an informed decision about your long-term goals for nurturing your child.

Breastfeeding is the perfect gift of love, security, and health all in one simple act. Just as your womb nourished your child for nine months, now your breasts are ready to continue that connection of food and nurturing for your baby. Just as your amniotic fluid acquired tastes and smells from your diet and your infant swallowed this while in the womb, breast milk also has flavours from your diet; and after birth, your baby continues to experience many new tastes. This is a gift that money can't buy. Whether you decide to breastfeed for a few weeks, months, or years, this is your first opportunity to give your baby a gift with benefits that will last a lifetime. Earlier we discussed your baby's need for connection; what better way to meet his many needs than to be held and breastfed?

In recent years, research has confirmed that breast milk is truly a unique food that cannot be duplicated. Formula is not equal to breast milk. The evidence of this fact became so overwhelming that in 1997 the American Academy of Pediatrics adopted a policy statement recommending that children receive breast milk for twelve months or more. The World Health Organisation recommendations on the priority of infant nutrition are in the following order:

1. mother's own milk directly from the breast

2. expressed mother's milk fed to infant another way

3. other human milk (from a milk bank)

4. infant formula

One of the outstanding benefits of human milk is that it is custom-made for each infant. Mothers with premature infants make milk that is specifically composed for their infant with extra antibodies and proteins. Breast milk contains not only carbohydrates, fats, and proteins but also has growth hormones and special substances that enhance visual and brain development, as well as antibodies to fight infection. Scientists are unable to put these valuable substances into formula. Studies have shown children who breastfeed have fewer instances of ear infections, diarrhoea, and upper respiratory infections. The advantages carry over into later periods in life. Adults who were breastfed have lower cholesterol and fewer occasions of heart disease. Studies have also shown that women who breastfeed have lower rates of breast cancer and cervical cancer. In addition to experiencing fewer common illnesses and diseases, breastfed children have higher IQs.

You may not have considered the financial value of this resource that your body makes at no cost to you. If you were to bottle-feed formula to your infant for a year, it may cost between $1,200 to $2,700, whereas human milk obtained by a doctor's prescription from a milk bank would cost about $36,000 for the same period! No wonder mothers call breast milk "liquid gold." Your body provides your baby this perfect diet absolutely free.

Normally, breastfeeding is a skill that is easy for you and your baby to learn. Mothers and babies have been doing this for thousands of years. As with any skill, like dancing or driving a car, the more you do it, the better you get at it. Getting through the first couple of weeks may seem natural or, at first, seem awkward, but given time, you and your baby will enjoy this special experience more and more.

During the first couple of days, your body has a small amount of early milk called colostrum. This is the time when your infant can practise latching on and sucking before the milk begins to increase in volume from teaspoons to ounces. Colostrum is an effective laxative that can help clear the meconium (baby's first stools) from your baby's system. It is also full of antibodies to protect your baby from illness. If your baby is sleepy and uninterested in eating, you can always express your colostrum onto a spoon and feed it to your baby to entice him to want to feed. Holding your baby skin-to-skin is another way for your baby to become interested in feeding. Studies show that the breast secretes a smell similar to amniotic fluid to attract the baby.

Learning a new skill is easier when someone is helping you. You didn't learn to drive a car by yourself. Remember to ask for help. Watching other mother's breastfeed before your baby is born will help you learn faster, too.

You may experience some breastfeeding challenges during the first week, but as you did during your pregnancy, keep a positive attitude toward breastfeeding. It soon becomes a gift to both mother and baby alike. If you experience discomfort, know that it is not a normal part of breastfeeding and indicates that you need attention. The earlier a problem is identified, the easier it is to solve. Lactation consultants and breastfeeding support volunteers are available in most communities. A supportive health-care provider or hospital staff will have information and can refer you to a breastfeeding expert in your area. Setting up your support system before your baby is born and learning about breastfeeding from knowledgeable sources like the La Leche League can minimise problems.

If problems do occur, there are two things that you can do while you are looking for help. First, maintain your milk supply. As long as you remove milk from the breast five to eight times a day, you will make more milk. If your baby cannot feed from the breast, remove milk with hand expression or use a breast pump. The second thing you need to do is feed your baby. You can use the milk you have expressed, or you may find that you need to supplement with formula until your supply increases. A baby who is gaining weight will be eager to learn to breastfeed. Support and timely "hands-on" help will create a positive learning environment for him.

It is important for people close to the mother to be emotionally supportive of her decision to breastfeed. Many fathers and grandparents today want to play an active role in caring for the new baby and wonder how they can be more involved if the baby is motherfed. There are many ways they can participate in other daily activities besides feeding. Walking, holding, rocking, and burping the baby after feeds can support the mother in these activities and allow the baby to get to know others in the family. While changing nappies may not be as appealing, it is another way for others to show they care! Baby's bath at the end of the day is a wonderful way for fathers to connect with their children.

Remember your reasons for learning about HypnoBirthing? You were looking for a birth experience that is calmer and safer for you and your baby—one that will give you more confidence than other experiences that your friends and relatives may have had in their birthings. The same is true with breastfeeding. Well-meaning acquaintances may have had difficulty breastfeeding because they could not find help or information when they needed it, but don't let that stop you from making this important decision for your baby. After the birth of your baby, Mother Nature assumes you will breastfeed and provides you with an abundance of milk. This is the time to go with breastfeeding and see how much you and your baby enjoy this special bond. It is a most special gift that you and your baby will surely appreciate, and it will build a bond that will last for a lifetime.

The Birth Afterglow

Together you bond in love
Each one defined as three;
All three connected as one . . .

A Celebration of Life

Much is said of the adjustments that parents of newly born infants must make in meeting the changes in schedules and the life tasks that are all of a sudden just there.

However, one doesn't often hear of the significant adjustments that your new little infant will be making as he emerges from the life of ease and security that he knew in his womb life and enters into the earthly environment.

During those months in which your baby has been developing within your womb, he's been comforted by the closeness and warmth of the wall of the membrane that softly caressed, soothed, and nestled him. Your baby has felt the gentle stimulation of the swirling waters, and he's been lulled by the subtle movement of your body. He has heard and felt the love that you offered as you talked and played together.

Birth has brought an abrupt ending to that safe, secure period of life within the womb. At the moment of birth, your baby emerged from his unencumbered world into a whole new series of experiences.

What your baby felt as he made his way into the world was a profusion of sensory encounters that can help make his transition easy or cause him to tremble, jerk, and cringe in fear. This experience can leave your baby with a birth memory that will affect his entire life, his personality, and his spirit.

The baby startled as he took that first breath on his own, felt air brushing across his skin, and bristled to the roughness of fabric used to rub the protective vernix from his body.

The manner in which you laboured and birthed, and the atmosphere into which your baby was born, should have offered the same love and care that you provided as you carried him. Only you can ensure that your baby's initial adjustment into his new surroundings is made as gentle as possible by planning and directing how his welcome will proceed.

Today's movies and television shows portray birth as comedic or traumatic; but no one realises the effect upon the emerging baby. The birthing environment following his emergence should have the same respect and calm as a place of worship. Great or humble, the decorum and protocol surrounding the birth of each and every baby should be conducted in a manner of reverence.

From the moment of birth, those first few seconds, minutes, hours, and weeks can be enormously important in shaping your baby's perception of what life is. This is his first lesson, and there should be a conscious effort on the part of all who are involved to ensure that it is a lesson that says his world is one of love, respect, and gentility.

Your baby's entrance is not always as genteel as we would like to see. As a result, the adjustments that he needs to make are enormous, but not all participants are cognizant of his worldly or his spiritual experience at this time. As parents you need to see that he is protected from the hustle and bustle that can exist in a birthing room after a baby is born. Voices should be subdued, and the room immediately returned to the soft lights and calm environment that existed prior to his birth.

At this time, assuming all is well, the only arms and hands that should hold your baby are yours and those of your partner. For some time, the baby needs to be sheltered from what could be a frightening experience of being introduced to the scent and the energy of others. Most hospitals today assure parents of at least an hour to become acquainted with their new baby before the onslaught of well-intentioned friends and family. All participants must keep in mind that these situations are frightening and disturbing to a newborn who is just getting accustomed to breathing and absorbing his new life outside of the womb. One hour is not nearly enough, one week is not enough. In some cultures parents and babies seclude themselves for as much as two to three weeks where their baby is kept in dimness and calmness, knowing only the soothing voices and gentle touches of his parents.

When parents kindly educate others in the family and close friends of what a traumatic time this is for a newborn baby, most will readily understand and honour the parents' explanation. Grandparents and friends can visit and observe and extend their well-wishes, but the baby should not be handed from one to the other until he is well on his way to accepting and adjusting to his new environment.

Responding to your baby's needs and learning that his cries are his way of communicating that he needs comforting and support are important. It is essential that he learns that he is accepted and that he is a loved and loving human being.

Some childbirth educators more affectionately call this special time a "babymoon." Much like a honeymoon, this is a time to get to know each other.

Because there is a considerable development continuing within your baby's brain and in her body even after birth is completed, it is important that you keep in mind the transitions that she is facing.

Some babies seem content in their new world, while others seem to experience the transition with difficulty. Allow your baby some time to adjust to her new life by making it as simple as her life in the womb as possible.

Your entire focus in these first few weeks should be on your baby's adjustment and not on hosting well-wishers. The privacy and the moments of exploring and getting acquainted are just as important now. You all need calm and peace and bonding as much as you did before your baby's arrival.

To begin with, minimise contact with the outside world. Simplify your daily life to meet your basic needs. Wear your pyjamas all day and order in food. This is not the time to have a constant stream of coworkers, friends, and relatives drop in. Guests, especially female, tend to want to hold new babies, but it needs to be remembered that babies are making a tremendous adjustment. They need to get accustomed to the scent and the touch of their parents and to become acclimated to their new surroundings.

Allow friends and relatives to visit only if they are bringing you a meal, want to do laundry, go shopping for you, or clean your house! Having these needs met makes the next leg of your journey into parenthood enjoyable and rewarding, and helps to create a transition into your new roles as parents and your infant's new role of going from pre-born to newborn.

Birth Preference Sheets

The following pages are copies of the worksheets that your HypnoBirthing practitioner will provide for your use in designing your birth preferences. It is a good idea to complete the Birth Preference Sheets prior to touring the facility you will use for your birthing. You may wish to discuss some of the items with the person conducting your tour.

This plan has been developed for use throughout the United States and in several foreign countries. For that reason, you will find items on the plan that may not apply to you or the facility at which you will birth. Several of the items that are listed have been adopted by most hospitals and staff long ago. However, many of the requests that are routinely honoured in some geographic areas are as yet unheard-of in other areas of this country and outside of the United States. You may skip these items, mark them N/A, or extract only those that apply to your own preferences.

Dear Health Care Provider:

My birthing companion and I have chosen you, our health care provider, and you, our birthing facility staff, as the people we want to attend us when our baby is born. We have chosen the HypnoBirthing® method of quiet, relaxed, natural birth. From everything we have heard from others, we truly believe that you will do your utmost to help us attain our wish for a joyous, memorable, and most satisfying natural birth.

The information that follows is a copy of our Birth Preferences. We have given careful consideration to each specific request in our plan, and we feel that it represents our wishes at this time. We realise that as labour ensues, we may choose to change our thinking and wish to feel free to do so.

We're looking forward to a normal pregnancy and birth and understand that these choices presume that this will be the case. Should a special circumstance arise that could cause us to deviate from our planned natural birth, we trust that you will provide us with a clear explanation of the special circumstance, the medical need for any procedure you may anticipate, and what options might be available. In such an event, please know that after we have had an explanation of the medical need and have had the opportunity to discuss the decision between ourselves, you will have our complete cooperation. In the absence of any special circumstance, we ask that the following requests be honoured.

Please attach these requests to my prenatal record. I will provide other copies for:

❑ Hospital admissions
❑ My midwife
❑ Birthing clinic staff

Please make this information known to any other physicians, nursing staff, or midwives who may be attending the birth should you not be attending us.

Signed: _____
　　　　　Parent(s)

Signed: _____
　　　　　Care Provider

Birth Preference Sheets

Mother's and Birth Companion's Names:

We have chosen you to be our care providers, and we thank you in advance for honouring our birthing preferences and assisting us in achieving a gentle and natural birth.

Welcoming our baby:

We are preparing for our baby's arrival with HypnoBirthing®, and we anticipate a calm, natural birth. We will be using special breathing techniques and relaxation, including self-hypnosis. My birth companion will be actively involved in our birthing. He/she has been fully prepared to support me in decisions and techniques regarding our baby's birth. Please include him/her in all discussions as labour advances. We ask for your understanding and accommodation to the requests outlined below, allowing our labour and birth to unfold as naturally as possible. These preferences are forwarded with the understanding that should an unexpected special circumstance arise, you will have our full cooperation after discussion and explanation. With this goal in mind, we list the following preferences:

Onset of labour:

❏ To allow labour to begin naturally unless induction by medical means is truly needed for the safety of my baby or me.

❏ To remain at home until labour is well established

Admission to hospital:

❏ To return home if labour is not well established at 4 cm to 6 cm

❏ To have birth companion ensure that mother maintains fluid intake and output

❏ To enjoy only intermittent foetal monitoring, unless medical indication requires otherwise

❏ To discuss my "comfort level," rather than a "level of pain" or being shown a pain scale

❏ To feel free to dim the room and have soft music playing

❏ To have bed rails lowered to encourage perinatal bonding

During Opening and Thinning:

❏ To feel free to walk, move about, and to find the most comfortable and effective positions

❏ To allow for an undisturbed rhythm and flow of natural labour with few or no vaginal exams

❏ To labour in tub if one is available—if not, to choose the shower

❏ To be relieved of blood pressure cuff and foetal monitor belts between readings

❏ To snack and drink as desired if labour is prolonged

❏ To forego medical interventions, including rupturing of membranes and augmentation, without clear medical need. Membranes to remain intact until baby is fully born.

❏ To use natural means before moving to intervention if baby requires more optimal repositioning

❏ To exercise patience if labour slows or rests, and use only natural means to stimulate labour if needed

❏ To have full explanation and discussion of medical need and alternatives before moving to intervention

During Descent:

❏ To assume a position of my choice, change position, or remain in a relaxed pose

❏ To breathe my baby down to crowning with prompts from only my birth companion

❏ To bear down only when my body is in surge, using the natural expulsive reflex

During Birth:

❏ To allow baby to emerge physiologically, free of assist unless needed

❏ To suction airway only if medically necessary

❏ To have father or mother receive baby once head and shoulders are born

❏ To allow time for the placenta to be released physiologically

❏ To use artificial oxytocin injection to prevent hemorrhage only if there is clear indication of need

For Baby:

❏ To dry or wipe baby gently with a soft fabric if necessary

❏ To have baby placed directly on mother's abdomen. Dad will join in.

❏ To allow cord pulsation to cease before cutting cord

❏ To allow baby to crawl to breast and self-attach for first feeding

❏ To apply prophylactic eye medication after family bonding time

❏ To use oral Vitamin K in multiple doses or delay Vitamin K injection

❏ To have baby remain with mother and birth companion at all times

We thank you in advance for your kind support and assistance in helping us meet our goal of a beautiful, natural birth.

About the Author

Marie (Mickey) Mongan, the former dean of a small women's college, is the Director of the HypnoBirthing Institute, located just outside the Capitol City of Concord, New Hampshire. Mongan brings to her hypnotherapy and HypnoBirthing classrooms over forty years of experience as a licensed counsellor and educator. She has taught at college level and has worked with adults in education in public and private sectors. Early in her career, Mongan received recognition when she was named one of five outstanding New Hampshire educators. She holds certification as an advanced clinical hypnotherapist, a hypno-anesthesiologist, and an instructor of hypnotherapy. She holds many awards for achievement in the field of hypnotherapy, including the National Guild of Hypnotists President's Award, and the much-coveted Charles Tebbetts award for her contribution to the understanding and acceptance of hypnotherapy within the medical field. She also is a recipient of the Plymouth State College Alumni Achievement Award and received a lifetime achievement award from the International Association of Counsellors and Therapists in 2013.

In the spring of 1992, Mongan travelled to Moscow as an American Diplomat with the Bridges for Peace Foundation, where she taught personnel management techniques to Russian women.

Mickey Mongan is the mother of four adult children, all born with the Dick-Read method on which the HypnoBirthing philosophy is based. Her practise has included group and individual work in a wide spectrum of therapy applications, in addition to the HypnoBirthing programme that she shares with you in this book.

Bibliography

Books

Barber, Joseph, Ph.D., and Cheri Adrian, Ph.D., Eds. *Psychological Approaches to the Management of Pain*. Levittown, Pa.: Brunner/Mazel, 1982.

Barstow, Anne Llewellyn. *Witchcraze*. San Francisco: Pandora, 1994.

Bieler, Henry G., M.D. *Food Is Your Best Medicine*. New York: Random House, 1965.

Birch, William G., M.D. *A Doctor Discusses Pregnancy*. Chicago: Budlong Press, 1988.

Blaustone, Jan. *The Joy of Parenthood*. Deephaven, Minn.: Meadowbrook Press, 1993.

Bolduc, Henry Leo. *Self Hypnosis: Creating Your Own Destiny*. Independence, Va.: Adventures into Time Publishers, 1992.

Bradley, Robert A., M.D. *Husband-Coached Childbirth*. New York: Bantam Books, 1996.

Capacchione, Lucia, and Sandra Bardsley. *Creating a Joyful Birth Experience*. New York: Fireside, 1994.

Carmack, Adrienne, MD. *Reclaiming My Birth Rights*. Adrienne Carmack/USA, 2014.

Carola, Robert, et al. *Human Anatomy and Physiology*. New York: McGraw-Hill Education, 1990.

Carpenter, Carl. *Hypno Kinesiology: A Holistic Approach to Healing*. New Delhi, India: Sterling Publishers, 2003.

Contey, Carrie, PhD., and Takikawa, Debby, DC. *CALMS-A Guide to Soothing Your Baby*. Hana Peace Works, 2007.

Chamberlain, David. *The Mind of Your Newborn Baby*. Berkeley, Calif.: North Atlantic Books, 1998.

Charpak, Nathalie. *Kangaroo Babies: A Different Way of Mothering*. Great Britain: Souvenir Press, 2006.

Curtis, Glade B., and Judith Schuler. *Your Pregnancy Week by Week*. Cambridge, Mass.: DeCapo Press, 2004.

Davis, Elizabeth, et al. Heart & Hands: *A Midwife's Guide to Pregnancy and Birth*. Berkeley, Calif.: Celestial Arts, 2004.

Dick-Read, Grantly, M.D. *Childbirth Without Fear*. London: Pinter & Martin Ltd., 2004.

Dunham, Carroll, et al. *Mamatoto: A Celebration of Birth*. New York: Viking-Penguin, 1992.

Dunstan, Priscilla. *Dunstan Baby Language*, 2006.

Dye, John H., M.D. *Easy Childbirth: Healthy Mother and Healthy Children*. Buffalo, N.Y.: J. H. Dye Medical Institute, 1891.

Ehrenreich, Barbara, and Deirdre English. *Witches, Midwives and Nurses*. New York: The Feminist Press, 2010.

Ellerbe, Helen. *The Dark Side of Christian History*. Berkeley, Calif.: Morningstar Books, 1995.

Gaskin, Ina May. *Spiritual Midwifery*. Summertown, Tenn.: Book Publishing Co., 2002.

Goer, Henci. *The Thinking Woman's Guide to a Better Birth*. New York: Perigree Books, 1999.

Goulding, Joane. *SleepTalk*. Pennon Publishing, 2004.

Hawk, Breck, R.N., midwife. *Hey! Who's Having This Baby, Anyway?* Phoenix, Ariz.: End Table Books, 2005.

Harper, Barbara, R.N. *Gentle Birth Choices*. Rochester, Vt.: Healing Arts Press, 1994.

Hoke, James H. *I Would If I Could and I Can*. Glendale, Calif.: Westwood Publishing Co., 1980.

Idarius, Betty, L.M., C. Hom. *The Homeopathic Children Manual*. Idarius Press, 2nd Edition, 1999.

Jones, Carl. *The Birth Partner's Handbook*. Deephaven, Minn.: Meadowbrook Press, 1989.

———. *Mind over Labor*. New York: Penguin Books, 1987.

Jordon, Brigitte. *Birth in Four Cultures*. Waveland Press, Inc., 1993.

Kerr, Mary Brandt. *The Joy of Pregnancy*. New York: Golden Apple Publishers, 1987.

Krasner, A.M., Ph.D. *The Wizard Within*. Irvine, Calif.: American Board of Hypnotherapy Press, 1990.

Kroger, William, M.D. *Childbirth with Hypnosis*. North Hollywood, Calif.: Wilshire Book Co., 1970.

Lazarev, Michael, M.D. *Sonatal*. Bloomsbury, N.J.: Infinite Potential, Inc., 1991.

Leboyer, Frederick. *Birth Without Violence*. Rochester, Vt.: Healing Arts Press, 2002.

Lennart, Righard. *Delivery Self-Attachment*. Sunland, Calif.: Geddes Productions, 1992.

Lesko, Wendy, and Matthew Lesko. *The Maternity Sourcebook*. New York: Warner Books, 1985.

Longacre, R.D., Ph.D., F.B.H.A. *Client-Centreed Hypnotherapy*. Dubuque, Iowa: Kendall/Hunt Publishing Co., 1995.

Losier, Michael J. *Law of Attraction*. Victoria, B.C., Canada: Michael Losier, 2003.

McCubbin, Jack H., M.D. *The Unborn Baby Book*. E.P. Dutton, 1987.

McCutcheon, Susan. *Natural Childbirth the Bradley Way*. New York: Plume, 1996.

Mitford, Jessica. *The American Way of Birth*. New York: E. P. Dutton, 1992.

Nathanielsz, Peter, M.D. *The Prenatal Prescription*. New York: HarperCollins Publishers, 2001.

Northrup, Christiane, M.D., Ph.D. *Women's Bodies, Women's Wisdom*. New York: Bantam Books, 2002.

Odent, Michel, M.D. *Birth Reborn*. Medford, N.J.: Birth Works Press, 1994.

O'Toole, Marie T., Ed. *Miller-Keane Encyclopedia and Dictionary of Medicine, Nursing and Allied Health*. Philadelphia, Pa.: W. B. Saunders Co., 2003.

Peterson, Gayle, Ph.D. *An Easier Childbirth*. Berkeley, Calif.: Shadow and Light Publications, 1993.

Schwartz, Leni. *Bonding Before Birth—A Guide to Becoming a Family*. Sigo Press, 1991.

Sears, William, M.D., and Martha Sears, R.N. *The Birth Book*. Boston, Mass.: Little, Brown, 1994.

Shanley, Laura Kaplan. *Unassisted Childbirth*. New York: Bergin & Garvey Paperback, 1994.

Simkin, Penny. *The Birth Partner*. Boston, Mass.: Harvard Common Press, 2001.

————, et al. *Pregnancy, Childbirth and the Newborn*. Deephaven, Minn.: Meadowbrook Press, 2001.

Stone, Merlin. *When God Was a Woman*. Orlando, Fla.: Harcourt Brace & Co., 1976.

Straus, Roger A., Ph.D., *Strategic Self-Hypnosis*. New York: Simon & Schuster, 2000.

Strong, Thomas H., Jr., M.D. *Expecting Trouble*. New York University Press, 2002.

Sutton, Jean, and Scott, Pauline. *Optimal Foetal Positioning*. Birth Concepts: New Zealand, 2nd Edition.

Thomas, Clayton L., Ed. *Taber's Cyclopedic Medical Dictionary*. Philadelphia, Pa.: F. A. Davis Co., 1997.

Vander, Arthur, et al. *Human Physiology*. New York: McGraw-Hill Publishing Co., 1997

Vaughn, Kathleen. *Safe Childbirth*. London: Bailliere, Tindall & Cox, 1937.

Verny, Thomas, M.D. *The Secret Life of the Unborn Child*. New York: Dell Publishing, 1981.

Weil, Andrew, M.D. *Spontaneous Healing*. New York: Ballantine Publishing Group. 1995.

Wessel, Helen. *The Joy of Natural Childbirth*. Bookmates International, Inc., 1994.

Wildner, Kim. *Mother's Intention: How Belief Shapes Birth*. Ludington, Mich.: Harbor & Hill Publishing, 2003.

Wirth, Frederick, M.D. *Prenatal Parenting*. New York: HarperCollins
   Publishers, 2001.

Worth, Jennifer. *Call the Midwife*. Phoenix, 2008.

IT GETS EASIER:

Surviving Twins During Their First Year

Tracey Egan

Nothing in your experience can prepare you for having twin, your new life plus two. Having twins is a unique experience. It is fun, busy, and, at times, overwhelming. It brings out an entire range of emotions: profound joy, overwhelming pride but also doubt and worry.

Tracey Egan guides the overwhelmed, and often exhausted, parents of twins through that crazy first year. Reassuringly comprehensive, *It Gets Easier* is an essential reference that will support and guide parents of multiple children through the myriad choices they have to make. Discover how to prepare in advance, accessible tips on coping with daily life, routines for feeding, teething and sleeping that suit your family's needs and how to preserve self-confidence in that hectic first year.

"A comprehensive guide for preparing for the arrival of twins ... but Tracey Egan's priority is to reassure and guide parents through until it does get easier."
'Easy Parenting'

It Gets Easier reassures as much as it advises because it really does get easier and easier, until one day you find yourself relaxing with a cup of tea while the twins are having a nap, and those crazy early weeks and months are a distant memory. It is a book for all mothers, not only mothers of multiple babies, as the ideal preparation for surviving the first year when parents need most help and reassurance.

"A unique perspective, focusing on the first year after birth ... The book is useful for all parents with lots of tips for surviving the first year."
'Practical Parenting'

KANGAROO BABIES:

A Different Way of Mothering

Nathalie Charpak

Kangaroo Mother Care was originally created in Third World countries where there is a shortage of incubators to help low-birth-weight-infants develop into healthy babies. The benefits of incubator care are simulated by a parent who keeps in almost continuous physical contact with the newborn baby. Babies are bound to their mothers, or other carers, in skin-to-skin contact and this physical contact regulates the babies' body temperature, and provides essential stimulation, as well as initiating bonding between baby and parents. This skin-to-skin contact keeps the baby warmer and calmer, as well as helping to regulate better breathing and a more stable heart-rate.

"A fantastic book . . . A must read for any parent new to the concept of Kangaroo Care." 'Little Bliss'

In this illustrated and practical guide to kangaroo mothering, Nathalie Charpak provides all mothers, and medical professionals, with an essential guide to an approach that will change the way mothers relate to newborn babies, and which will improve the way hospitals treat premature babies. More than thirty countries follow the Kangaroo Mother Care method and now any mother can use this method to begin bonding with their baby immediately, and the baby can begin life in the most healthy and nurturing way possible.

"This lively, highly readable little book is for everyone who works with maternity and neonatal services . . . a heartening, honest, practical, non-nonsense guide to a method of care that will appeal to most people for sensible reasons."
'Infant Journal'

Available in ebook and as a paperback edition

The FitMama Method™:

Your complete guide to confidence and fitness for birth

Marie Behenna

Giving birth is the single most challenging physical activity the majority of women will face in their lifetime.

So why not prepare for it by training and exercising, by toning your body so that you can approach labour and delivery with calm confidence, free of the anxiety and tension that complicate so many births. *The FitMama™ Method: Your Complete Guide to Confidence and Fitness for Birth* has been based on Marie Behenna's own experience of pregnancy and birth and her work as a personal trainer. It encompasses not only exercise but also advice on diet, nutrition, posture, recovery and general wellbeing.

"A brilliant, no-nonsense resource for women looking for advice on staying active throughout their pregnancies." 'Bodyfit'

Marie Behenna has been preparing pregnant women for birth, both physically and mentally, for over twenty years, and by following her unique programme of gentle exercises you'll find that you gain confidence and knowledge as your pregnancy progresses. *The FitMama™ Method* will guide you through the physiological changes of pregnancy, the choices you can make during labour and delivery, and how to ensure a full and swift recovery. You won't need complicated equipment, and you can perform the exercises in the privacy of your own home.

"Aims to help pregnant women and new mums look after their bodies . . . Easy to read and reassuring . . . An excellent way to be informed."
Parents in Touch